STRONG
THE NEW FIT

FADI MALOUF

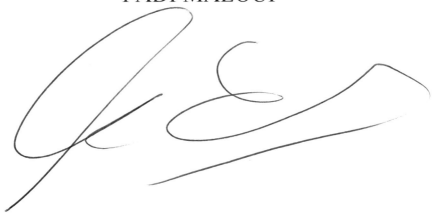

Body By Fadi Online

Learn more about Fadi Malouf and visit Body By Fadi at: www.fadimalouf.com become part of the online wellness community, gain access to our amazing Workout Anywhere Anytime solutions, receive fitness and nutrition support, coaching, life mentoring, updates and many additional wellness resources.

Tell Us Your Story

I love transformation stories. By giving you my life journey in Strong The New Fit I hope you will feel inspired and empowered after reading my triumphs and struggles. If you have a transformation story that you would like to share, then send it to me! Please know that your story may land on my website or on one of our next books! support@fadimalouf.com

For my father Nabil

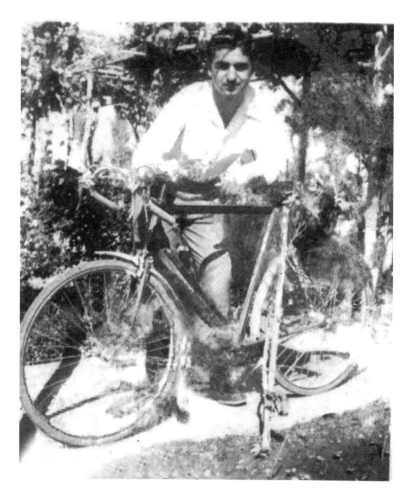

Contents

STRONG *The New Fit* will teach you how to use your inner and physical strengths to be healthy in body, clear in thought, vital and active, as you have fun and realize your dreams.

Fadi learns a painful lesson that will alter the course of his life.

Make the positive choices that will help you become your possibilities.

Fadi faces a difficult transition to a new life in Georgia.

Let your own Core Values guide your actions.

Fadi struggles for respect as he experiences difficult physical challenges.

An exploration of the nutritional keys to optimum health.

Introduction

We've all been there. It's that moment from which we can't hide. We initiate an action, or speak our mind, and in doing so cross a point of no return. Julius Caesar's army did it in 49 BC, engaging in an act of insurrection by crossing the shallow, muddy waters of the river Rubicon, in northeastern Italy. P.T.G. Beauregard did it when he authorized a 10-inch mortar round be fired against Fort Sumter in Charleston Harbor on an April morning in 1861 – the first shot of the American Civil War.

In your own community, a young man, overwhelmed with love, drops to his knee to profess undying love for his girlfriend, asking her to become his wife. At the moment he presents his ring, he has crossed the Rubicon; fired the first round. It's done. Win or lose, there is no turning back.

The risks can be worth it. Caesar won. He cast his die as his enemies fled in fear, releasing him of consequences for his infraction. Beauregard survived his four-year war, lived to tell about it, and died quietly in his sleep 22 years later in New Orleans. But his region fared poorly and suffered great losses.

As for the young man who laid open his heart and proposed? She said "Yes!"

Life is like that. There are many things we can't control and some things we can. Your decisions, and the actions you initiate, can have far reaching effects. And sometimes, whether you intended to or not, you may feel you've crossed that *point of no return.*

You may *believe* there's no hope for losing those unwanted pounds, or no chance you could restore your cholesterol or blood pressure to safe levels. Are you struggling to build a meaningful career following your college graduation, or perhaps you're trying to rebound from job loss. These are the times you need strength.

It may seem incongruous, but strength does not come from winning. Your struggles develop your strength. When you pass through hardship and consciously decide not to surrender, you become strong.

That's when you learn to recondition your thoughts. You can learn and apply proven ways to make your choices succeed for you. In the pages of *STRONG / The New Fit*, you'll discover that points of no return don't always mean there's no way out. There is hope. You haven't crossed the Rubicon, even if you've overlooked your health for years. You *can* reframe your lifestyle and transform your fitness. When you harness the courage to act on your dreams, you can produce results that change your life forever.

I struggled mightily through the story you are about to read. I can testify through hard-earned lessons that strength means facing your truths, pushing through obstacles, and getting on with life despite constraints and encumbrances.

As you learn my story, you'll meet a shy immigrant child, pulled from a tiny developing country in the Middle East and dropped unceremoniously into a 1970s small town America. This child, wise for his years but still naive, struggled to find his place, hampered by language barriers and nearly incapable of reading and writing.

As the story unfolds, you'll discover how a developing young man dealt with physical deficiencies and devastating injuries, bullying, learning disabilities, failures, and loss. You'll experience his adjustments within a dynamic culture, and ponder his struggles to find and define love.

My life could have had many endings, tragic or incomplete, but I am a man who chose to stand steadfastly through the blows of change. I discovered the fortitude to face my giants and juggle sacrifices, continuously pushing for progress. When my own pillars of support broke down, I became the support others needed.

In the immediacy of my greatest loss, as a teenager, I began to transform my life. Tapping into the wisdom and strength of trusted mentors, I began developing my once frail body into levels unimagined. As I came to redefine my own fitness, I discovered a form of conditioning that breaks down the walls of negative thought.

The foundation for this conditioning started with physical work, as I acted on my desire to remake my body to its highest level of fitness. Pushing myself even harder than my brother and trainers pushed me; I soon discovered truths about the mental and social conditioning necessary to support the physical effort. As I developed my form, my mind became sharper, my thoughts clearer, and I translated my health and newfound focus into financial success. I started to realize the results I once only dreamed of knowing, and it was due to reframing my thoughts.

I had mastered *Strong*, a complete and balanced life made possible by *The New Fit*, my system for defining what matters most, and intentionally acting on specific goals that create better results for my life.

I began simply as a curious boy from Jordan, with language deficiencies and a frame prone to breakage, who overcame physical and mental barriers, and fought through pain and confusion. I found the capacity to keep my head up and move forward, no matter how tough things got. And in doing so, I remade myself into an international body building champion, elite fitness trainer, actor, model, public speaker, and entrepreneur.

As you learn more about my life, and discover my proven system for remaking your own, I hope you will be inspired. *STRONG / The New Fit* will teach you how to break down the walls that have held you back from being the complete person you are meant to be.

STRONG / The New Fit is part biography and part self-improvement. As a whole, this book offers a practical guide to a safe and natural weight management and lifestyle program built upon five key components: Nutrition, Resistance Training, Cardiovascular Training, Accountability, and Motivation.

The narrative chapters in *STRONG* recount my stories, focusing on poignant experiences and lessons that shaped my life and molded my philosophies on fitness and life success. I hope you will connect with my emotional and psychological stamina, which has allowed me to transform my personal and professional being into excellence, in a healthy and natural way, free from steroids and other drugs.

In alternating chapters, I share details of *The New Fit*, providing practical methods to help you reach your optimum fitness level. As your health improves, your energy increases, your mind sharpens, and you can develop other key aspects of your life. You will learn how your efforts can result in a life of continuous improvement, teeming with possibilities. When you learn to apply my Work Life Balance to your own life, you will fully realize the meaning of *STRONG / The New Fit*.

Within some chapters are *Fadi Features*, related short stories or simple how-tos, which offer further instruction or inspiration. A *STRONG / The New Fit* Discussion Guide follows Chapter 16. This guide offers thought-provoking questions inspired by each chapter. Book Club members, business groups, students, or individuals can benefit from the Discussion Guide, as they reflect and share on the ideas and concepts of *STRONG / The New Fit*.

So let's get started on a journey that may very well change your life. My story begins along the rocky slopes of north-western Jordan, near a city built on seven hills.

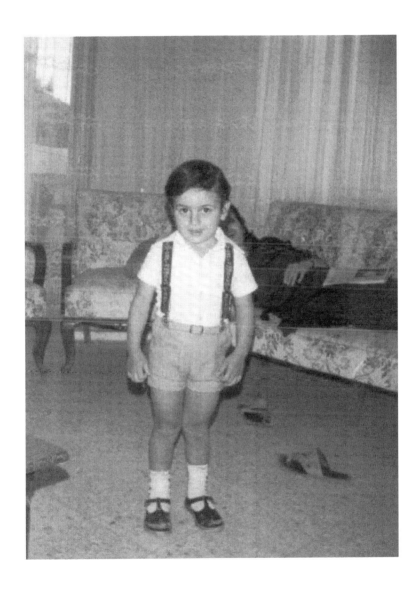

Chapter 1
Head Up

I squirmed in my chair, becoming increasingly restless. Even as my mother Salwa placed a glazed clay bowl of steaming soup before me, I barely allowed myself to savor the smells of roasted shallots, fresh carrots, noodles, and chicken. Our neighbors from the small house next door, built of concrete and just a tall man's length from our own home, had gathered with my family, the Maloufs, for a late afternoon meal. On nearby couches, the men of the group, including my father Nabil, shared stories of the day as they sipped sweetened Arabic coffee, careful to avoid the finely ground bean sludge that settles at the bottom of each cup.

Salwa's soup, gently seasoned with minced garlic cloves, cayenne pepper, and the bitter but alluring cumin, would be just the first course. I knew that when the empty soup bowls were cleared, my mother would place before our family and friends the "upside down" *maglooba*, a favorite casserole of Jordanians, featuring chicken, potatoes, basmati rice, eggplant, and seasonings of cinnamon, nutmeg, salt, and black pepper. I found it fun, almost magical in my 7-year-old eyes, to watch my mother place a large platter on top of the pot where the maglooba was cooking, the bottom of the platter facing up. She would hold tightly onto the pot, and quickly flip the pot and platter over so that the platter would shift to the bottom. Flipping it upside down would bring all the juices and delicacies to the top. Small dishes of plain yogurt and chopped *salata* - tomatoes and cucumbers mixed with a little salt and lemon juice - would complete the main course.

But on this June afternoon in 1983, I was distracted. I was far less interested in sitting through a meal than I was trying out a seemingly new British-made bicycle I had received for my birthday a few days earlier. The bike, a Raleigh Grifter, now leaned against the side of our house, gleaming in the bright sun, which baked this neighborhood of Amman, at the edge of the Great Rift Valley, in 96 degrees of searing heat. If it could talk, I was sure the Grifter would be saying, "Fadi, ride me. Come now and let's play."

The gravel lane that fronted my home was perfect for a bike like this – straight for as long as I could see looking north, and southward curving slightly towards my grandmother's house, with occasional mounds of dirt along the shoulders that could make great ramps for jumps. A paved highway, one I understood never to cross, ran parallel to the gravel road, separated by a rutted, loosely packed open field.

The Grifter was beautiful in my eyes: Blaze Blue exterior, with handlebar mounted twist grips and tire mud guards; the rear mud guard several centimeters longer than the front. The elongated saddle dipped in the middle. Handlebar foam, stretching from grip to grip, and a three-speed hub gear made this bicycle almost irresistible.

So irresistible in fact, that I hurried through this meal as fast as I could, careful not to eat so fast that I attracted the disapproval of my parents. The last thing I wanted was to be forbidden from going outside after the meal.

Although I had not yet ridden my bicycle, or any

other bicycle for that matter, I felt confident I could manage. It did not come with training wheels, but that mattered little. As a toddler, I had watched with curiosity as my older brothers, Baseem and Basil, had ridden bicycles, and I felt sure that when my time came – and it most assuredly had arrived now – I would be able to mount and ride.

Since receiving my bicycle, I had patiently waited for the time when my father Nabil would be available to help teach *me* the proper way to mount and ride a bicycle. My oldest brother Baseem was now gone; sent to California in the United States a few years earlier for an education that Nabil and Salwa hoped would provide him a stable and successful life. My father had told me he would teach me how to ride my bike this week.

"Until you are taught to ride, leave it where it is. We will practice soon."

As the adults continued to talk, and shared a dessert of locally grown oranges, the neighboring children and I slipped out of the house. I could hear the adults laughing through an open window. My friends began to chase one another, running into their own yard and back and forth to a small building used for storage. I moved straight to the Grifter; like a magnet pulled to steel.

Two trucks along the paved highway barreled past the houses. Many of the trucks that regularly passed by belonged to the Royal Jordanian Land Force – army vehicles traveling to and from a nearby base. The roar of the diesel engines and the dust these massive transports stirred up each time they passed were as common to our small enclave of neighbors as the sandstone rocks that littered the dirt lane in front of our homes.

I wiped my hands onto my white t-shirt and checked front and back to make sure my shirt was tucked into my blue shorts. I looked down at my black sneakers, to make sure my laces were tied. I paused to listen, to see if I could still hear my parents talking. It was quiet, and then I thought I heard my mother say, "Where is Fadi?" I made no audible response. Perhaps I imagined hearing her voice? Still I did not move. More adult conversation ensued, and I could stand it no longer. I reached to my bicycle and with a hand on each twist grip, began to maneuver it from the house to the gravel lane.

I looked toward my playmates. They had gathered in a circle, sitting on the ground dozens of meters away. They were happily engaged in a game of rock, paper, scissors, and shooter.

I was now on the gravel lane, at the edge of the field. I again looked across at my friends. I looked toward my house. It was time to ride my Grifter. *Fadi – Conqueror of the Wheels!* As I held tightly to the handle bars, I climbed onto the frame, straddling each side, and settled quickly into the saddle. No problem.

I thought about what I had seen others do. I put my left foot onto a pedal, and adjusted it down, so that it was closer to the ground. Then I placed my other foot on my right pedal. I pushed with my right foot and that pedal dropped forward and down, forcing the left pedal back and up again. My bike started to move forward.

Feeling unsure and less than confident I moved only a couple of feet forward, then dropped my left foot to the ground again. I tried again and moved a little more. Again…and then one more time. I got off my bicycle, and stood beside it, looking again toward my house. Did anyone notice me out in the lane with my bike? I rolled it to the field separating the house from the highway, so as not to draw attention.

My shirt was sticking to my chest, blotched with perspiration in the intense heat. My hands and arms were beaded with sweat.

"One more time."

I decided that on this attempt, I would mount quickly, and begin pedaling right away, instead of trying to balance myself on the bike and then attempting to pedal it. I would try to make it move forward in one fluid motion, like a nomad leaping onto a camel, then leaning backward in the saddle and holding on for dear life.

In an awkward motion, I jumped aboard my bicycle and, holding tight to the hand grips, looked down at the pedals and started pushing my legs as hard as I could. The Grifter began rolling – awkwardly – bumping across the field. I was certainly not in control, but I was not yet out of control either.

Less than a quarter mile up the road, on the highway, a 10-ton army lorry, with dual wheels on the rear axles, moved steadily at 50 miles per hour, headed toward its base a few miles south. A brown-eyed soldier in the shotgun seat stared out and observed what appeared to be a dark-haired child on a bicycle wobbling across a field toward the highway. He alerts his driver, and points, who glances in that direction, and curses in alarm.

By this time, I spot the large military truck, with an open bed covered by a frame and canvas, headed on the highway in my direction. Although I remained in the field beside the highway, my bicycle had quickly shifted from a slow wobble, as I first tried to manage it, and had now accelerated to an uncontrollable shake - *a death wobble.* The whole bike felt very light and frail as I gripped the bicycle more tightly.

I wobbled, and shook violently....within 10 meters of the truck, I fell, landed on my right knee and right arm, and ground to a halt, my senses now as aware and alert as a prowling cat. The lorry, without braking, now passed me, belching out smoke as the young soldier in the shotgun seat stared down and then back at me as the truck roared onward.

My t-shirt was stretched and dirty from the grinding fall; my right knee, scraped and bleeding slightly, and the sting in my right shoulder, pink and tender, burned as if on fire.

I sat up, but remained on the ground beside my bike, my back towards my house. Time seemed to move in slow motion. What seemed like several minutes, perhaps was only seconds. I dared not cry out.

I looked at my knee, a raw abrasion, and prepared to lift myself up.

"Fadi. Stand up. Pick up the bike."

I froze in fear. I wanted to leave my bike and run, but I was too stunned. I winced again from the sting on my shoulder.

"Father, I'm sorry…." I now looked up at Nabil, standing over me. My eyes watered.

Nabil helped me stand up and collected my bicycle, which didn't appear to be damaged, save the absence of pristine newness that disappears after something is broken in for the first time.

The two of us walked toward the house. By now my mother was located outside of the front of the house, a small towel clutched in her right hand.

"FADI! What were YOU doing?!"

My stomach felt like it had been punched. I stood awkwardly now beside my bike, practically leaning on it as I held it with one hand. My father and I had reached the dirt lane near the house.

Nabil examined my injuries. He determined them to be too minor to stop.

"Let's try again. Get on and ride."

I looked up at my father, and then remounted the now broken in Grifter. My father steadied the frame as I began to push down the left pedal.

I tried to ride again, but the gravel rocks dotting the lane appeared as big as sand cats. I looked down to attempt to navigate over the uneven terrain, but bumped a jagged stone, fell left, and pounded the ground. My left elbow ached. My right foot twisted awkwardly.

"Get back on the bicycle."

I looked at my father. I wanted to protest, but I knew that was not an option.

I stood up and collected my bike. I remounted, adjusted my stance, and maneuvered the handlebars, realizing a slight wobble and then stumbled. Ugh.

"I'll walk near you, Fadi." My father waited for me to attempt another ride.

I now awkwardly straddled the bicycle, both feet on the ground, and waited, expecting my father to steady it as I prepared to push off.

"I'll walk beside you," said my father, not touching the machine. "You pedal and ride."

I lurched forward, pedaling as steady as I could, trying to navigate around the rocks I saw in my path. I swayed from side to side and fell over to my left, away from the side where my father was standing.

Dust spiraled upward when my hip hit the ground.

Both my father and I were sweating profusely.

"Too many rocks," I told my father. "It hurts to fall."

"Try again, Fadi. I'll walk beside you."

A small tear rolled down my right cheek, snaking a

path through my dirt stained face. I did not utter another sound as I wiped the tear off with the back of my left hand.

My elbow and knee stung. I straddled the bicycle yet again.

"Ride now, Fadi. I'll be beside you."

I began to pedal. I focused on the rocks and dips, determined to steer my front wheel around them. I missed a large piece of sandstone, but the back tire rolled over another, I started to shake.

Suddenly a sharp tug pulled my straight black hair. My father yanked my hair at the back of my head near my lower right ear. My head lifted up, as I felt a slight burning sensation...surprised, but eyes wide open.

"Head up. Don't focus on the bigger rocks. Concentrate on where you want to be."

I tried again to ride, this time keeping my eyes up, watching the road ahead as I began to pedal, one revolution at a time. I was moving forward. Time and again I pedaled forward, picking up speed and momentum. The rocks began to seem like pebbles.

They were always there, those rocks. I discovered that each time I thought about them or when I looked down, I would hit them. When I kept my head up, and I focused on where I was going -- the lane straight ahead and I could ride like the wind.

This was an important lesson to me. I did not fear to try, but I could not succeed without guidance and a painful lesson in focus. Whether I realized it or not, at the impressionable age of seven, on a dusty lane at the outskirts of Amman, I had gained my first understanding of *STRONG*.

Chapter 2
Moving Forward

At an early age, along hot dusty roads in a developing country smaller geographically than the state of Indiana, I first began to understand the concept of goals and focus. I began to realize that any obstacle in life can be overcome if you keep your head up and continue to move forward. It's often not easy. There are bumps, and falls, and occasional crashes, but you learn something valuable every time you fall. And most importantly, you recover and adjust, and keep moving forward.

In recent years, after many setbacks, and during times of challenge, I'm inspired by a cinematic conversation, a perspective on life shared by an aging boxer to his adult son. Fictional boxing legend Rocky Balboa spoke earnestly to his son Robert, in the film Rocky VI.

"You, me or nobody is going to hit as hard as life. But it ain't about how hard you hit, it is about how hard you can get hit and keep moving forward, how much can you take and keep moving forward. That's how winning is done!"

I relate these lessons so often to health and fitness. You, my friend, by taking the time to read my story and the truths I've learned over 37 years, have started down a road that leads to a fit, healthy body and a life without limits. I know beyond a doubt, and I want to help you understand (to paraphrase tennis legend Arthur Ashe's observations on success), that *health* is a journey, not a destination.

In *STRONG / The New Fit*, you will discover how much we have in common. We may not have traveled the same journey, our destinations may not match in detail, but we both have experienced challenges, hardships, and even tragedy in our lives, despite any differences in age or gender that may exist.

My story may not mirror your own. The people who have influenced us, or supported us, or even disappointed us, may not be the same. The names and faces of the loved ones we have lost, who left their marks on our lives but are now gone, will likely be different. But our journeys are not dissimilar.

I was not always a world-class bodybuilder, leading personal fitness trainer, successful entrepreneur, model, actor, international speaker, and results expert. These are roles in my life that emerged and developed as a result of determinedly moving forward despite obstacles in my journey.

I was once a small shy boy, pulled from my country of origin during preadolescence, and transplanted to a place where I could not speak the language. As a young immigrant with literacy barriers to overcome, I often struggled in school, and endured bullying during the challenging years when puberty was changing my body and my mindset. I faced devastating physical injuries from sports, a refuge to which I turned to build friendships, injuries which could have blocked me from becoming the man I am today. I had to find the strength to grow up faster than I expected while still in high school, after losing one of the most influential persons in my life.

These are storylines of my own life, which you will experience as you continue through *STRONG / The New Fit*. While I share my story in hopes of inspiring you as you move forward in your own, I will also offer you specific personal tools to live your dreams, enjoy the journey as you travel, and become your possibilities.

The first step on the road to a sound and fit body is learning to make the right decisions in your nutritional and exercise choices. This step means understanding that these nutrition and workout choices *become* a lifestyle that never ends.

The day you consciously or unconsciously step off this road is the day your weight will begin to increase and your health starts to decline. Live out those correct choices, and marvel as your health improves, your confidence builds; you begin to think more clearly, and enjoy greater energy. As this happens, you will be increasingly motivated to act on your dreams, put more play into your life, and have fun achieving your milestone goals. You'll become your potential.

I applaud you as you move forward in this journey of fitness, a journey that will change your body and your life forever. This positive choice, your commitment to *yourself*, will pay off every day for the rest of your life.

As a child, I had to decide how I would live my life, as it changed and evolved. I like to think that when confronted with options, I made good choices. Perhaps that's true in some cases. But the reality is, I sometimes had no options, and what choices existed, were sometimes made for me.

Chapter 3

Adaptations

A tall administrator led me into a brightly lit classroom. I stopped just inside the door and looked around. Eight- and nine-year-old boys and girls sat around four different tables, pulling dried elbow noodles through red yarn. Their teacher leaned over one group, assisting with a scissors exercise.

Across the room and near a window, a nylon rope stretched across the room from two walls. A chain of construction paper cut into colorful strips stapled together hung from the makeshift clothesline. Each paper link featured words, written in black crayon, scrawled on the outside. Below the window stood a small bookshelf, packed with well-worn paperbacks, many of which bore dog-eared covers. Wedged together were two or three copies of some older titles, such as *Charlotte's Web* and *Runaway Ralph.*

"Boys and girls, please give me your attention," announced the tall man in blue slacks and white shirt, accented by a skinny blue-and-gold necktie. He waited for the students to set aside their projects and turn to look toward me. "This is Fadi Malouf. He is going to join your class, beginning today."

One thick-haired boy wearing a red and white rugby shirt and dirtied Wrangler jeans, looked over at me and chuckled, but not too loud to attract his teacher's glaring eye.

"Fatty? That's his name?" he said to his friend beside him. "He doesn't look fat to me."

I glanced at the boy, but I didn't smile or frown. Even if I could have clearly heard him, I wouldn't have understood a word he said. I processed all I saw and heard in Arabic, not understanding the cues and words those around me. A wave of loneliness, edging on terror, washed over me.

I viewed my family's move to the United States in the summer of 1985 as more of an adventure than a permanent relocation. My parents Nabil and Salwa had sent my brother Baseem, their oldest son, to California six years earlier. They wanted all of their children to have access to the educational opportunities that living in America could offer. As parents of a daughter and three sons, my parents also were not keen on the mandatory military service expected of Jordanian males when they turned 18.

That summer, just weeks after the Hashemite Kingdom of Jordan celebrated its 39th anniversary as an independent nation, I turned nine. I was excited about going to America, although I really didn't understand where it was I would live.

As my mother sat in our home's enclosed patio for the last time, the final boxes packed and taped, I stood and walked to a favorite balcony, sealed with glass windows. The rocky field outside was very familiar and comforting, the place where I had defined my young life.

I lingered a moment more, then looked back at my mother and stated, flatly, "We're coming back to Amman."

"No, you are not coming back," my mother Salwa told me, pausing in reflection. "You're moving permanently. That's it."

Stone Mountain, the largest exposed mass of granite in the world, is located in DeKalb County, about 15 miles northeast of downtown Atlanta. Before 1800, Native Americans met at the mountain and held ceremonies and other spiritual gatherings. European settlers first discovered Stone Mountain and its natural beauty in the late 17th Century, and many more Europeans moved into that area in the early 19th Century. In the 1850s, the mammoth rock was already popular with tourists from the Atlanta area. By 1970, state dignitaries dedicated a massive Confederate memorial carved into one side, and attractions such as a steam engine-driven train, local festivals, and a laser light show, which debuted in the 1980s, created a tourist attraction that draws millions each year. A small town at the base of the mountain bears the same name.

When my family, the Maloufs, moved to Stone Mountain in the mid-1980s, there were very few Middle Eastern families living in the area. I soon learned that in Stone Mountain, Georgia I was a minority, one of very few like me.

As I became acclimated to American schools and customs, I remained extremely self-conscious, acutely aware of differences in culture and language. I thought and spoke in Arabic, which made attempts to read and write in English that much more agonizing. Given even a simple poem to read aloud, I would drone, hesitate, and torture words.

In time, my deficiencies caught up with me. No educator apparently doubted my potential for learning; each recognized my intelligence. But the learning barriers I faced proved too much my first year in an American school, and I, dismayed, learned I would repeat the Fourth Grade. "It will help you catch up to your peers," my teacher told me.

Down, battling feelings of failure, I eventually stiffened my resolve and vowed that next time, I'd do better.

From the time I could walk, I had always enjoyed being outdoors, spending sun-drenched hours running, and chasing, and wrestling with friends as I grew into a fit boy, lean and sinewy.

In elementary school, on playgrounds and ball fields in the shadow of Stone Mountain, I began to notice my increasing physical abilities. Still quiet and self-conscious in the classroom, I became more animated and extroverted when outdoors, playing with friends. I also discovered in myself a competitive tendency, fueled by a need for perfection.

Some days during recess, I would line up to race, typically a sprint across the playground against other boys in my grade level. I ran hard, often winning my races by several yards. But sometimes I'd fall behind a bigger kid, and when it became clear I would not win, I simply wanted to quit. Second place was not good enough for me. I needed to win. Anything short of victory angered me, and intense emotions would well up inside, ready to erupt.

By middle school, my Arabic gave way to English, as I learned to speak and communicate much more effectively. With increasing confidence, I befriended classmates across different social groups, all of whom appreciated my carefree sense of humor and athletic acumen. Life for me as an adolescent took an upward trajectory, yet there were still some doubts. Reading and writing, the Achilles Heel of my academic experience, still lingered in that gray area of "needs improvement."

As I entered my early teens, I began growing, edging upward toward my eventual height of 73 inches, even rising four inches in 12 months. To acquaintances, I grew strikingly handsome -- tall and lean, with brown hair and deep brown eyes, marked with an engaging smile. Yet I remained quiet and soft spoken, not one to draw attention to myself. Some of my shyness may have stemmed from a personal crisis in confidence. At home, my mother forbade me from answering the telephone. "Don't pick up that phone," she would tell me when it rang. "You don't know what you're doing."

During these formative years, sports continued to provide me an outlet for my energies. While searching for a personal identity, I discovered the value of affirmation, of positive self-talk. When feeling nervous, or inadequate in some way, I learned to tell myself, "I'm stronger today than yesterday, and I'll be stronger tomorrow."

Looking ahead to high school, I started to believe my own words of inspiration and my confidence grew. I was coming into my own.

Chapter 4
Persistence

Every new day, regardless of what may have transpired on the preceding day, I wake up expecting blessings and anticipating positive results of my intended actions during the next 24 hours. It's an inner motivation, a drive to continuously improve and to help others become their possibilities that pushes this expectation of success and goodwill. I anticipate positive results because I know that, no matter what happens, I will persist.

It is persistence, the ability to maintain action regardless of personal feelings that gives you the strength to move forward even when you feel like quitting. Motivation by itself does not produce positive results. It is the actions you continually take, prompted by your motivation, which yields measureable results time and again.

I recall a tale about three frogs, sitting on a log in a pond. Three frogs are balanced on the log, several feet off shore, and two frogs decide to jump.

How many frogs are left on the log? You may have answered "one," but that's not correct. Two frogs decided to jump, but neither actually jumped. Three frogs remain on the log.

This is how it is with any decision you make. You can decide to be a fit person, one who is active and vital and enjoys the rewards of a clean mind and healthy body.

But wanting that lifestyle and doing it are not the same. You can't just decide in your head that you are *going* to do it. You've got to frame what is most important to you – your core values -- and then decide that you are going to commit to a healthy lifestyle. You've got to "jump off that log" and then work on it every day.

You can sit on the log for a long time and say, "I'm going to lose 20 pounds." Eventually, if those pounds are to disappear, you'll have to jump, and as you land you can begin the actions that will result in that weight loss and restored fitness. If you keep taking action, you'll eventually get results, and those results will motivate you to take more action.

Keep-in-mind that like a child's game of tug-o-war, you'll likely experience some back and forth. You'll pull hard, and your opponents will begrudgingly inch closer to the line that spells your victory, then they rally and yank the rope and you stall. When your motivation wanes, such as reaching a temporary plateau in your weight loss, your persistence prompts you to keep taking action until your motivation returns. The end result: You keep accumulating desired results. You pull the stubborn opposition across the victory line. You win.

My Core Values for a Healthy Lifestyle

A key to my successes is crafting and adhering to Core Values, a concept I adapted from Steven Covey's influential book, *The Seven Habits of Highly Effective People*. My values frame my daily decisions. When I face challenges, or reflect on how to address a perplexing issue, or re-evaluate my goals in relation to my standing at a moment in time, my Core Values keep me moving in the right direction.

Each of you probably has a set of basic Core Values, whether or not you have written them or if are even aware of them. I hope you have written them down as a form of understanding and commitment. You have roles in your life, just as I do.

In my life roles, I am a loving son, a supportive brother, an inspiring leader, a businessman, fitness expert, health icon, financial giver, passionate lover, great friend, and playful mentor. You have your own roles, and how you define and live your roles are no less important to you and your friends and loved ones.

We all need to clearly define key elements of our personas: Our Purpose, our Mission, our Roles, and importantly, our Core Values. Understanding who we are, and who we strive to be, gives us the motivation we need to take intentional actions, and drives us to persist when things don't always go as planned.

We are all a work in progress, with many unknowns in our paths, but we need to know who we are, for what we stand, and how we plan to get there. "Think positively about yourself, keep your thoughts and your actions clean, [and] ask God who made you to keep on remaking you," wrote inspirational author Norman Vincent Peale. I love the part in that quote about asking God to keep on remaking you. Your Core Values are your blueprint for your continuous remake. These Core Values guide your decisions and ultimately help you reach the results that define you and who you wish to be.

I strongly encourage you to reflect on your life and write down your set of Core Values. As you do, create categories for different types of Core Values, and write down Action Items that you will follow to live out these Values.

I share my personal Core Values below, as a model for you as you draft your own. My Core Values will help you better understand my life's priorities, what I deem most important in life, who I strive to be, and how I plan to act on these Values. These Core Values link closely to my business philosophy – summarized by *Dream, Play, Be* (which you will learn about later) -- and also my personal Mission and my Purpose.

As a businessman, founder of My Fitness Solution, MFS Academy and Body By Fadi, I am always cognizant that when I am not in my personal space and time, I will ALWAYS, ALWAYS be listening to what is IMPORTANT and VALUED in others. I encourage you to do the same.

Before proceeding towards our Core Values consider the following as you progress through each day.

- Watch your thoughts for they become words.
- Choose words for they become actions.
- Understand your actions, for they become habits.
- Study your habits, for they will become your character.
- Develop your character, for it becomes your destiny.

This simple acronym has proven to be very helpful:

W — Watch your Words.
A — Watch your Actions.
T — Watch your Thoughts.
C — Watch your Companions.
H — Watch your Habits.

"The best way to predict the future is to create it."
                                        Peter Drucker

As Peter Drucker states, you are your best avenue for creating success in your life. Make the decision to change, track your decision to change and stick with your decision to change and believe that you will change.

FADI MALOUF'S CORE VALUES

Feel free to use my Core Value personal development work as an example to help establish your Core Values. If you do, an exciting life changing mind and body "Reboot" will occur. Once you are "re-booted" your internal compass will align with your goals and dreams.

Thought - Motivation by Purpose = **Take Action** Change before you must!

Theme - Share your Dreams – Play, keeping life fun & Be your possibility!

Time - When I am not in my personal space and time, I ALWAYS, ALWAYS listen to what is IMPORTANT and VALUED in others. "A dime a day will keep the doctor away".

My Purpose - Making a Difference.

My Mission - To be a man of my word, a bold leader, inspiration for growth, respect and love for every family, friend, and partner.

My Roles: I am a...

- Loving Son - Reach out to mom, ask her what she needs or just perform a random act for her that she would see of value.
- Supporting Brother - Reach out to my siblings asking them what they need or perform random acts for them that they would see of value.
- Inspiring Leader - Lead by example, relate to individual's struggles, request to help them and follow through with my commitments. Speak often authentically and powerfully.
- Business Man - Driven, persuasive, strong negotiation skills, and follow ethical business protocols.
- Fitness Expert - Stay updated to current fitness trends and practice what I preach.
- Health Icon - Look healthy and be healthier.
- Financial Giver - Contribute 15% + of my time and money to worthy charities.
- Passionate Lover - Spice it up and put my heart into it to my loved one.
- Great Friend - Listen and make myself available even if its business related.
- Playful Mentor - Entertain my niece, nephews and other kids while inspiring them to learn and take action.

My Core Values

At the core of my belief is that "Your Words Have Power" so, I have learned over time to use them wisely.

My understanding of this truth became very clear upon discovering and reading *"Power Vs. Force"* written by Dr. David Hawkins.

Dr. Hawkins book presents the results of millions of tests conducted on thousands of subjects over a period of 20 years. This testing has proved to be replicable and most basic requirements of scientific enquiry. Hawkins used kinesiological testing to create a map of human consciousness and a profile of the human condition.

The book illustrates a logarithmic scale of consciousness against which things can be calibrated with 1 being the lowest possible state of consciousness and 1,000 representing the highest possible state of human consciousness achievable.

Check out *"Power Vs. Force"* to learn which words are your power words and which words are negative words. And discover which state of mind is your "Power" center!

Faith/Authenticity – Believing in a higher power, practicing active faith and being a servant and contribution to society first. Honesty is my freedom. (DREAM)

ACTION ITEMS: Visit all levels of consciousness, Pray/Meditate Daily, Be Honest and Share my Dreams!

Integrity/Clear Communication – Words and deeds match up, I am who I am, no matter where I am or who I am with. I honor my word. (PLAY)

ACTION ITEMS: Follow through and stay in communication. Focus on OUTCOME or keep the end in mind.

Family – Being with my family and communities, both quality and quantity of time. Be aware of who I am in each community and know what I stand for.

ACTION ITEMS: Reach out to each family member once a week devoting service, quality time, gifts or an empowering affirmation/acknowledgement (write thank you cards). Use the 5 Love Languages.

Growth – Investing in lifelong learning and self-education. High value to enlightenment, wisdom and loyalty to creating lifelong relationships with people for abundance in health and wealth. Build business for decades to come.

ACTION ITEMS: Journal daily, attend school/class, build financial security and create opportunities that last a lifetime and history. ONLY SHARE powerful and cutting edge knowledge with TRUE LIFE PARTNERS!

Passion – Intense emotion, excitement, boundless enthusiasm and just pure love. I will love and share the ebbs and the flows of my life.

ACTION ITEMS: Share passionately on the moment, when I speak, educate and open up to near and dear loved ones.

Fitness – Spiritually, mentally, physically, emotionally, financially and socially fit; I condition to optimal well-being to accomplish all possibilities that I create.

ACTION ITEMS: Pray/affirm beliefs, exercise hard, study for outcome, write vividly, be compassionate, invest wisely, and share authentically.

Gratefulness/Joy – Acknowledge life as it is and accept what "is". Sharing thanks, laughter and leaving myself and other inspired right away!! (BE)

ACTION ITEMS: Celebrate all wins, acknowledge people, be thankful and journal daily, acknowledge and share my blessings, keep people smiling and share on the moment!

Rules to Success

Calling it – If I am not acting on my beliefs and commitments which soon delivers my character the opportunity is yours and mine.

Little Voice – Mastery author Blair Singer noted, "One of the most important sales of all, in any part of your life, is selling you to you!"

You have to believe in your Core Values, because the intent is to live out those values. As you write your Core Values, you have got to believe in them; you have to be sold on them. Your own chart of Core Values may be similar to mine, but it is okay if it isn't. These values need to reflect exactly what *you* believe, what *you* desire out of life, and how *you* intend to follow these values (your action items). Having Core Values without Action Items is like the frog that sits on the log and intends to jump off but has no plan for doing it. If you are not living your Core Values, then have a trusted friend or loved one call you on it. Accountability to others for the choices you make is a powerful motivator and can kickstart you towards living the life you intended.

Affirmations – We all need affirmations, small words or phrases that we write or recite to ourselves to motivate us to action or help us persist. Some of my personal affirmations:

- I am obsessed about what's best for other as well as what's best for me.
- I am better today than yesterday and great tomorrow. - Fadi Malouf
- I am great.
- I am wonderful.
- I am smart.
- I am a money magnet.
- I have more to give.
- I have money and time to contribute.
- I will give 110% at everything I do.
- Be not the slave of your emotions but a master of empowerment through self expression. - Fadi Malouf
- Be the best that I can.
- Be honest with self and others.
- Be proactive instead of reactive.
- Be authentic.
- Be patient.
- Be present.
- I am my habits. My habits are me.
- Man is disturbed not by things, but by his opinion of things.

- Both partners must take responsibility for the outcome.
- Learning is a gift even if the teacher is pain.
- Dream wildly, write vividly, and WORK your deepest desires. - Fadi Malouf
- People value my expertise and are willing to pay top dollar for it because it makes a difference in their life and transforms - Fadi Malouf
- One of the most important sales of all, in any part of your life, is selling you to you! -- Blair Singer
- Contribute to society with money, time or both!
- Transform society through health and fitness.
- Believe in yourself, if you don't, no one else will. -- Fadi Malouf
- Take the time and enjoy watching things in your life, grow and evolve. -- Fadi Malouf
- Have Faith and believe in others.
- Think before you say or do anything.
- You only lie when you're afraid.
- Find the source.
- The key to success is playing to people's strengths.
- True communication is the response that you receive.
- When it's all said and done relationships are what it's all about Together for Life. -- Fadi Malouf
- Whenever you're in conflict with someone, there is one factor that can make the difference between DAMAGING your relationship and DEEPENING it. That factor is ATTITUDE.
- It's better to LOVE and be heartbroken, then to NEVER love. -- Unknown
- Change before you must. -- Earl Suttle
- "Profits are BETTER than wages." -- JIM ROHN
- "Money isn't everything, but it ranks right up there with Oxygen." -- ZIG ZIGLAR

- "You can get anything you want out of life, as long as you help enough other people get what they want." -- ZIG ZIGLAR
- "When you win the rat race, you're still a rat."
- "Whether you think you can, or think you can't, you're always right." -- Henry Ford
- "If a man empties his purse into his head, no one can take it from him." -- BENJAMIN FRANKLIN
- "I'm not BIG on history, but I'm BIG on making history!" -- KETAN V. HIRANI "
- To have something you've never had, you've got to do something you've never done!"-- UNKNOWN
- "Make everyday count, rather than count every day!" -- KETAN V. HIRANI
- PROGRESS - "Coming together is a beginning. Keeping together is progress. Working together is success." -- Henry Ford
- PROGRESS - "It doesn't matter which side of the fence you get off on sometimes. What matters most is getting off. You cannot make progress without making decisions." -- Jim Rohn
- "Readers are leaders."
- "No income becomes a bad outcomes." -- Robert Allen
- "Long after what you said or did, they will remember how you made them FEEL."
- "It's true... My DREAM is beyond me! My PURPOSE and the PEOPLE in my life will lead me to that DREAM." -- Fadi Malouf
- Feel the BURN and be ACCOMPLISHED!!!
- Dream wildly, write vividly and WORK your deepest desires.

Business Priorities - Boulders First

1. Mastering Sales $30k/month - ACTION: Schedule 15 sales appointment per week
2. Mastering Financial and P&L Statements - ACTION: Review weekly, monthly, quarterly & annually using QuickBooks. Use 50/30/20 financial ratios.
3. Mastering Public Speaking - ACTION: Speaking once week 10 people, monthly 30 people, quarterly 60 people, and annually 120 people.
4. Building a Champion Fitness Professional Team - ACTION: 5 Remote Coaches
5. Publish Strong - ACTION: Market online and develop partnerships.
6. 500 active virtual accounts and 20k transformed by 2015 - ACTION: Use systems and empower individuals by following their PASSION and building their BEST.
7. 15 month travel around the world with inspiring documentation - ACTION: Schedule travel opportunities and document with video.

Guideline to Business Success

1. Income must ALWAYS exceed Expenses.
2. Collect payments on time.
3. Take care of your clients.
4. Take care of your employees and the people who work with you.

Use 50/30/20 financial ratios: 50% Operations / 30% Marketing / 20% Growth

Those are it! My Core Values! Let *your* Core Values guide you. Make them visible and keep them in the forefront of your thoughts and decision-making. Let these values guide your actions, and use affirmations to keep yourself motivated and honest. If you intend to take actions that don't comply with your Core Values, reconsider before you act. You only lie, to others or to yourself, when you are afraid. But why be afraid when you're living with a set of positive Core Values? Document your dreams and share those dreams with everyone, because you never know who the next person might be who will partner with you to make a difference.

Chapter 5

Becoming

Lean track athletes were milling around the interior of the oval track, some chatting sporadically, but most lost in their own thoughts. Several sat throughout the grass, leaning gingerly into themselves as they stretched their calves and quadriceps. Coaches busily emptied water bottles from duffle bags and set up portable tents. A few athletes warmed up for their upcoming heats, jogging around the green space to force more blood into their leg muscles as their heart rates gradually elevated.

I was a sophomore athlete among the runners engaged in warm-ups. As I stopped to retie my Reeboks, I glanced up at a competitor, whose physical features momentarily sent my thoughts back to Jordan, during my second and third grade school years. My mind flashbacked to Reshia, a classmate whose name meant "like a feather." Reshia was lanky and loose-jointed, light on his feet and lightning quick.

In Amman, Reshia and I raced often, both of us sprinting as hard as we could, running with sheer abandon, refusing to give in. Reshia naturally was fast, with blood like a cheetah, but what set him apart from other boys who raced me was his iron will. He wanted to win as bad as I did, and often he outlasted. Of all the boys in my school in Amman, Reshia became my nemesis -- the only one who could beat me in a footrace.

Brought back to the present when a coach called my name, I walked toward the track with some of my Redan High teammates. Our next event would be a 440-yard relay. Four boys would each run a quarter-mile, and the first three would pass a baton to a teammate.

I felt strong that morning. I was loose and focused, and expected to run well. Coach placed me as the first runner. It would be important to get a strong push off the block and to run the curves well. My baton exchange to my second runner, who was taller than me and good on the straight-aways, would need to be flawless. I looked around to see if the boy who had reminded him of Reshia was in my relay race. He wasn't, and that was good. I didn't need any distractions.

I pushed off hard at the starting gun, forcing myself forward with the energy burst of a diesel-electric locomotive. Quickly I felt the presence of competitors along my periphery, but my focus narrowed on creating space as I powered forward. With each foot strike my knee flexed slightly, bending naturally at impact.

As I gained momentum, I straightened my torso and back, running upright now, ensuring that my hips, my center of gravity, carried me straight ahead. Knowing the baton exchange was near, I became irritated, burning to put more space between me and the rival six yards behind me. Leaning in, my torso hunched in slightly, perhaps too much, causing my pelvis to tilt forward. The actions placed pressure on my lower back, throwing my lower body out of alignment.

I groaned as my ischium bone, on the right side of my pelvis, fractured under the pressure of sudden muscle contractions. A hard yank of the hamstring muscle, where it latched onto the ischium, ripped off a piece of the bone, dropping me to the ground. Even as a burning sensation rolled through my midsection, I clenched the baton, looking up the track as my competition sprinted past. My race was over, and me the track runner, swollen and bruised, would not walk again for six months.

In the ensuing years, I learned more about my body than at any time prior to high school. Tests on my bones were troubling, showing them less dense and more brittle than would be expected of an active young man. Exercise triggers force on the bones that increase density, which makes them sturdier and helps protect against breakages. I had always been active, playing sports and outdoor games, but it appeared I lacked calcium. My body, hungry for more calcium to maintain nerve and muscle function, was using up the stores of calcium in my bones.

In many parts of the world, goat's milk is consumed much more than cow's milk. Goats are cheaper to maintain and require less pasture space and resources than dairy cows. My mother used goat's milk, and occasionally, forms of powdered milk. I felt the milk was either too thick or too thin, and I refused to drink it. Over time, my body lacked sufficient calcium. My bones suffered as a result.

By the time I was a senior and had transferred to Brookwood High, I discovered a type of low fat milk, rich in calcium, which had a consistency I could tolerate. I worked diligently in the weight room, developing my physique, and was learning so much about how the body responds to nutrition and strength training that I often argued with my high school weight coaches about the best exercises.

My bone density problem had disappeared, never to return. The pelvis fracture was not my first broken bone. A neighborhood bully delivered the first. During my thirteenth summer, long before my physical transformation in the gym, I started palling around with a pair of twin brothers, who lived down the street. I got along well with one of the twins, who was easy going. The other twin, short-tempered and intense, liked to bully other kids, especially the younger ones. Perhaps my quiet nature made me appear weak in the eyes of a bully, but one fall afternoon Bully (the mean twin) punched me in the back left side of my jaw, fracturing it in two places. Doctors wired my jaw tight, and I was still sipping juices from a straw at Christmas.

Basil, my older brother, advised me to seek revenge on the bully twin. "Go to him, and stand up for yourself," he told me.

Still wired at the mouth, I approached the Bully, determined to see justice done. Without uttering a word, I punched him in the chest, took a step back, and waited. Bully stared hard at me but didn't move. I kicked him in the stomach, turned, and ran, sprinting at a pace fast enough to leave Reshia in the dust.

As I fled, sheer panic flushed through me, and I looked back to see Bully chasing me on his twin brother's scooter. Bully was gaining ground on me. My prospects for safe refuge appeared dim. I barely made it through my own front door.

It seemed that every time I stood up for myself, I'd get beat up again. I found myself in that awkward period of adolescence, where hormones and teen angst rule. And, as the youngest neighborhood kid, I felt that I lacked respect. The older boys looked down on me; the older girls didn't notice.

I might have folded, and accepted my lowly status. No, despite the risks, I would continue to stand up for myself until I earned the respect I deserved. Where some viewed me as weak, I would prove myself to be Strong.

Chapter 6
Discoveries

When I lead nutrition-themed seminars, my participants often seem surprised when I tell them that 80 percent of being fit is mastering your nutrition. "As much as 80 percent of reaching an ideal body weight, with low body fat and high energy levels, is mastering what you eat, when you eat it, and how much of it you eat," I tell them.

"What?" some will inevitably ask, "If I'm working hard in the gym three or four days a week, don't I have the right to eat what I please?" Their assumption is that if you exercise hard enough, and often enough, you can eat whatever you want.

Yes, you have the *right* to eat what you want, including a lot of junk foods and processed heat-and-eat meals. Those foods aren't going to give your body what it needs. What you get is lots of salt, sugar, and fat in your body. A standard supermarket diet of salt, sugar and fat stimulate you to eat more than you need.

If you exercise constantly, like an obsessed hamster on a wheel, but don't eat a balanced, natural diet, you might look decent but you won't know ideal health. If you eat nothing but natural foods, but fail to exercise, you'll look bad, despite the types of foods you consume. "Exercise is king. Nutrition is queen," noted fitness pioneer Jack LaLanne. "Put them together and you've got a kingdom."

Make no mistake: Exercise is the catalyst for achieving health. Regular exercise increases circulation throughout your body, which drives all of your key body systems. Your circulation makes everything work as it is supposed to: Your skin, hair, digestion, elimination, and your sex life. Your nutrition provides your body the proper energy it needs to perform its necessary functions.

Fine Tuning Your Engine

Think about your automobile. If you make plans to drive your car for hundreds of miles to a vacation destination, you begin your trip with faith that the vehicle's engine and the structural frame will take you all the way. And to insure your car operates properly, you have to give it the proper fuel (oil and gasoline) along the way.

As you travel down the interstate, you'll encounter cars of all types. You will pass cars that are fairly new, but their owners don't take care of them. Those cars will start running poorly long before they should. Then you'll find cars that are decades old and still run like new. It's all about how the owner takes care of his car.

The kind of fuel you put into your car makes all the difference, too. An economy model may be able to run on any brand of gasoline, but a fine-tuned sports car requires premium.

Protein, such is found in fish and egg whites, is an essential nutrient (fuel) for any athlete. The right amount of protein in your diet is the best way to maximize your body's efficiency. Protein should be at least a quarter of an athlete's caloric intake per day, preferably closer to 40 percent. An athlete who works out on a regular basis will use that protein to stimulate the growth of muscle mass. Just as that well maintained and adequately fueled car will transport you to your destination, protein supplies the power for your body. It contains the kinds of nutrients, vitamins, and amino acids that energize and maintain muscle.

Eat like a bodybuilder to build lean muscle, which increases your metabolism and burns fat, to achieve and maintain a healthy weight. The basic idea is to balance proteins (about 40 percent of calories consumed), with carbohydrates (40 percent) and fat (20 percent). Each meal that you consume should have calories coming from proteins, carbohydrates, and fat.

Let's think about Jenna, a 42-year-old woman accustomed to eating five small meals throughout each day. During a mid-day lunch, Jenna meets a friend and consumes a non-typical meal consisting of 90 percent carbohydrates, five percent fat, and five percent protein. Jenna's thinking, "Oh, a low fat meal...this has got to be OK."

Jenna's 300-calorie lunch with her friend calorically mirrored that of the typical lunches she prepared, designed to align closer to 40 percent protein, 40 percent carbs, and 20 percent fats. Yet, Jenna's body digested the high carbohydrate lunch much faster, and she was soon hungry again, eager to satisfy her appetite. True, Jenna's body received about 300 calories from both lunches, but after digesting the high carbohydrate meal, her body prepared to store a percentage of the carbs as fat.

Frozen vegetables are generally fresher than "fresh" vegetables, as they are more likely to have been cut and frozen immediately out of the fields, thus avoiding preservatives to keep them looking fresher longer. Stay away from processed foods, the kinds of boxed and packaged meals your grandmother would not have recognized as real food. Those processed products may have extended shelf lives, but they are also full of fats, sugars, sodium, and preservatives that will extend your waistline, too.

Healthy eating is like putting the right kind of fuel in a car, but a car that you can never trade in. You can trade in a used car for a newer model, but you only get one body. Don't be someone who takes better care of their cars than themselves.

Fat Loss Formula 5/3/12

Now that you know what to eat it is also important to know when to eat. Fat Loss Formula 5/3/12 is your fat loss success formula: Eat 5 meals a day every 3 hours with a 12 hour fast between your last meal of the day and your first meal of the day.

This formula is not only good for fat burning but those seeking muscular gain can also benefit from eating 5 or 6 meals every day.

The following are a few reasons to eat 5 or 6 meals each day.

- Speeds up metabolism.
- Diminishes the desire to overeat.
- Puts less stress on your colon.
- Easier for your body to digest.
- Stabilize blood sugar levels.

The following tips will help you maintain Fat Loss Formula 5/3/12.

- Use a timer: your watch, smart phone, tablet, computer or other timer and set it to beep every 3 hours. Eat when it tells you to eat.
- Pre cook and pre package your food and keep it on hand.
- Carry easy to eat foods everywhere you go: Boiled eggs, healthy supplements, fruits and vegetables are good examples.

Resistance Train to Boost Metabolism

While what you eat is a key component of ultimate fitness, the types of exercises you do to build muscle and raise metabolism make a huge difference on how fast you can burn fat and keep it off. I'm often asked, "What's most effective for burning fat: running or weight training?"

Resistance training is the one thing that we do that elevates our metabolism for hours after a workout. Cardiovascular workouts are also effective and necessary. Running three or four times a week for 20-30 minutes can help burn fat, but after an hour of running, your metabolism is only elevated for less than an hour before returning to its normal levels.

Gaining lean muscle mass through weight resistance training literally will help raise your metabolism permanently. Strength training exercises, such as weightlifting, are important because they help counteract muscle loss associated with aging. This happens because weight lifting is actually breaking down muscle tissue and rebuilding it back stronger. Muscle tissue burns more calories than fat tissue does, so building muscle mass is a key factor in weight loss. When your metabolism remains elevated, your body is primed to burn off your fat.

Protein and Blood Sugar Levels

Beta-cells are tiny special cells scattered throughout your pancreas, an organ located under your stomach. These beta-cells produce insulin, store it within the cell as little granules, and release it into the blood stream at appropriate times.

If you are a healthy person who has not eaten in a while, these beta-cells release a small amount of insulin into the blood stream throughout the day and night in the form of very small pulses every few minutes. This is called "basal insulin release."

Your body needs to maintain this steady supply of insulin. It allows the cells of the body to utilize blood sugar even if some time has passed since your last meal.

Your insulin level communicates to your liver as well. As your insulin level drops, your liver is signaled that your blood sugar is getting low. The liver knows it is time to add more glucose.

When this happens, the liver converts the carbohydrates it has stored, (known as glycogen) into glucose, and dumps it into the blood stream. This influx of glucose into the blood steam raises the blood sugar back to its normal level.

If a person has exhausted their glycogen stores, as can happen on a nutrition plan low in carbohydrates, the liver converts protein into glucose. The glucose from protein is created in response to a low level of insulin in the blood.

The protein can come from protein you eat or, if you are not eating sufficient protein, from your body's own muscles. That is why you can lose significant amounts of muscle mass if you don't get enough protein in your nutrition plan.

To prevent your blood sugar from rising above and below acceptable levels, meals should be eaten every two to four hours, or approximately three hours apart. Five small meals per day – planned to balance proteins, carbohydrates, and fat -- is ideal. Your first meal should be within one hour of waking up, and a great breakfast choice is a slow-acting carbohydrate, like stone rolled oats. This pattern -- eating small balanced meals every three hours, supported by eight hours sleep each night, will keep your body satisfied and rested, and operating at its optimum efficiency.

Half Your Body Weight

All of us understand our biological need for water. Our body is estimated to be 70 percent water. Blood is mostly water, and our muscles, lungs, and brain all contain a lot of water. Water regulates body temperature and makes it possible for nutrients to travel to our organs and tissues. We need water to remove waste, and to transport oxygen to our cells. Water protects our joints and organs.

Can drinking water help us lose weight? German researchers in 2004 reported that water consumption increases the rate at which people burn calories. The

German study reported that after drinking approximately ½ liter of water, their research subjects' metabolic rate (the rate at which calories are burned) increased by 30 percent for both men and women within 10 to 40 minutes. Experts agree that more research is merited.

I subscribe to the belief that you can estimate the amount of water you need by taking your weight in pounds and dividing that number in half. That gives you the number of ounces of water you should drink each day.

Let's think about a Kyle, a 28-year-old man who weighs 220 pounds, and wishes to lose 55 pounds. Kyle is trying. He exercises daily for 30 minutes, does not drink alcohol, and is generally healthy. For maximum health benefits and to assist with his desired weight loss, Kyle should drink 110-113 fluid ounces of water today (approximately 3.3 liters, or 3.5 quarts). Since Kyle is active, he should drink another eight ounces of water for every 20 minutes he exercises.

Your water needs vary based on other factors. Pregnant women or women who breastfeed may have different water needs. The same is true if you live in a hot, dry climate, at a high altitude, or if you became sick with fever or diarrhea.

If Kyle eats a healthy diet, which would include a properly balanced portion of protein (beans, lean poultry, fish), carbohydrates (whole grains, fresh vegetables and fruits), and fat (almonds, flax seeds, olive oil), he could expect that about 20 percent of his water may come from the foods he eats. So, with his healthy meals, he could drink about 100 ounces of water over a day's time. With his healthy diet, Kyle could drink about 90 ounces of water today, or 2.6 liters. As the great Chef Julia Childs noted, "Water is the most neglected nutrient in your diet, but one of the most vital."

If you find it difficult to measure and track how much water you consume, then plan to drink about 10 glasses of water each day, or two glasses with each of five small meals. Water is the obvious source for your daily fluid needs, but other good beverages include teas, such as herbal and green teas.

I limit the use of dairy products to my clients trying to lose weight or keep off weight they've lost. A non-dairy product, soy milk (as long as it does not contain added sugar) or almond milk, is preferable to cow's milk. In small amounts, I allow for some plain, non-fat Greek yogurt, for its muscle-supporting protein and its "good" bacteria for your digestive tract. Cottage cheese has casein protein, which digests more slowly than other types of protein, supplying your muscles with a steady stream of amino acids while you sleep. Blending together these and other ingredients into Smoothies is an enjoyable way to bring them into your daily nutrition.

Soy milk is made from beans, and therefore contains about nine times less saturated fat than cow's milk. Saturated fat is one of the leading contributors to heart disease. Another heart-stopper is cholesterol, known to clog arteries. Cholesterol free soy milk also has 10 times as many fatty acids, and lower LDL, or "bad" cholesterol. You'll also find plenty of phytochemicals in soy milk, which provides additional heart protection.

Creating An Energy Deficit

When we talk about metabolism, we mean the natural body process by which your body converts what you eat and drink into energy. A complex biochemical process combines oxygen with the calories in the food and beverages you consume to release the energy your body needs to function. Such energy is needed for breathing, circulating blood, growing and repairing cells, and adjusting hormone levels.

All of us have a basal metabolic rate (BMR), which is measured by the number of calories your body uses to carry out these basic functions that keep you alive and healthy. We often call this BMR our *metabolism*.

Your individual basal metabolic rate varies from others for several reasons. As you get older, the amount of muscle tends to decrease and fat accounts for more of your weight. This can slow down the rate at which you burn calories. If you have a larger body type, or have more muscle, you will burn up more calories, even at rest. Men burn more calories than women of the same age and weight, since those men typically will have less body fat and more muscle regardless of fitness levels.

Your basal metabolic rate accounts for about 60 to 75 percent of the calories you burn every day. Another 10 percent of the calories you use are consumed in digesting, absorbing, transporting and storing the food you eat. The remaining 15 to 30 percent of the calories your body burns daily is due to your physical activity and exercise. Any physical movement, from cleaning the garage, to running, or pushing a stroller at the park, will burn calories. Make intentional calorie-burning exercises, such as resistance training, become part of each day. If you aren't moving to raise your heart rate and stimulate your metabolism, you aren't burning the extra unwanted calories.

Weight gain is the result of eating more calories than you burn. To lose weight, you need to create an *energy deficit*. When you eat fewer calories, or increase the number of calories you burn through physical activity, or both, you'll create an energy deficit. That means you are burning more calories than you eat. And that's when your unwanted extra pounds start to disappear.

Chapter 7

Finding Love

Kerrie

Until I met Kerri, I had rarely thought much about colors. Sure, I appreciated colorful flower beds bordering suburban lawns and sometimes artwork stood out when bold hues jumped off the canvas. I had once heard about colors having different meanings, such as red symbolizing courage and orange inspiring endurance.

But as a high school senior, I had other more important thoughts to occupy my mind. I attended classes, practiced football, trained daily in the gym and generally enjoyed the standing that seniors earn after nearly 13 years of school. Reflecting on color schemes ranked low in my thoughts.

Not so for Kerri, a stunning brunette who simply adored the color yellow. Kerri had other interests too, including helping to choreograph halftime routines featuring flag waving teams of dancers and gymnasts. And I, who had worked myself into the best shape of my life, soon caught the admiring eye of Kerri.

It didn't hurt that I played football, the most popular sport in the state, on a team known to dominate its rivals. I realized that playing the game gave me added prestige in the eyes of girls like Kerri.

Kerri surrounded herself with yellow - the color of optimism, enlightenment and happiness. Perhaps she knew that yellow stimulates our minds and nervous systems, activates our memory and encourages creative thought. Or, maybe Kerri just liked the color for its warm, bright shades. Her reasons were likely personal, but she was clearly attached.

Whatever the attraction, I soon learned that if I dated Kerri, I took the world of yellow with her. Kerri loved Tweetie Bird, the long-lashed canary with speech impediments made famous in classic *Merrie Melodies* cartoons. Kerri had a different outfit for every day, usually accentuating shades of yellow. I once discovered Kerri with 100 yellow balloons on her birthday.

One evening, towards the end of one of our first dates, I found myself standing outside Kerri's yellow Volkswagen Beetle with her at my side. A first quarter moon hung in the sky concealing half its form in shadow. The Beetle's driver's window was down with its radio tuned to WSTR 94.1 FM, an Atlanta pop music station. Kerri and I chatted and spoke about an upcoming pep rally. An autumn chill dampened the air and Kerri fastened the uppermost buttons of her yellow cardigan sweater.

I put my arm over Kerri's shoulder, offering to keep her warm.

As we quietly talked, familiar chords wafted into our consciousnes and the unmistakable voice of Tina Turner began to croon...*You must understand that the touch of your hand makes my pulse react...that it's only the thrill of boy meeting girl, opposites attract...*

Kerri turned toward me, looking into my eyes. Neither of us spoke a word. Kerri dropped her gaze and her eyelids to half mast. Then slowly she looked back up at me, offering me a small welcoming smile.

It's physical...only logical...you must try to ignore that it means more than that...

I looked into Kerri's eyes, reaching around her waist to gently draw her toward me. Kerri reached up and twined her arms around my neck, lightly playing with my hair. Our lips, slightly parted, finally met, as I felt a flutter deep within my stomach – the unforgettable rush of a first kiss.

A few seconds later, without speaking a word, our eyes met again and she smiled. I hugged Kerri, gently, as she nestled her head on my shoulder. *Oh what's love got to do, got to do with it? ...What's love but a second hand emotion? ...What's love got to do, got to do with it?*

A few weeks later I decided to do something I had never done before. I decided to open up my heart completely. I would meet Kerri after school and tell her I loved her.

This act of courage, verbalizing my love for Kerri, was unique for me. I was raised to show love through service to others, not speak words of affection. In sharing my feelings, I risked the possibility of love unrequited, enduring the pain of discovering that my strong romantic feelings for Kerri might not be returned.

Perhaps, I had reasoned, this was a one-sided affair, a relationship I had built up in *my* mind as special, but one Kerri simply viewed as platonic. If I told her how I felt, would she love me back, or would she back away -

rejecting me outright and crushing my self-esteem?

Kerri smiled when I laid my heart open before her. She hugged me and kissed my right cheek. Although I didn't hear the words I had hoped from her, I decided it was going well and followed up by asking her to be my Prom date.

"I'd like that," Kerri replied. Then told me she'd like her ex-boyfriend, a member of the marching band, to attend the Prom with us. Kerri preferred a date for three: herself, me, and "the ex".

That marked the beginning of the end of our relationship. My puppy love experienced growing pains, and Kerri became the first girl to break my forlorn heart. Years later, I still remember how perplexed I felt, the confusion of it all.

I've never figured it out.

Amber
Up until Amber I had never crossed the trust line between client and trainer.

But the attraction was unmistakable, unshakeable. The kind of attraction that was much stronger than base pheromones. You know, those pheromones that make it difficult to know the difference between true love and that primal call of the wild.

As her trainer I was the consummate professional and our sessions were amazing and full of fitness fire. But it was in the "off" times when we spoke of non fitness items that the relationship started to show. I remember well how I would often spill my coffee, trip over myself and lose my speech capabilities in her presence after our training sessions were over.

Our love was impassioned and full of fire just like our training sessions. We enjoyed life to its fullest and had that "spark" and those roller coaster moments that dizzied the world around us. We were "Ken and Barbie". We were "soul mates". All of our friends knew it and loved us for it!

I loved Amber but the way I showed my love was not what Amber needed. I grew up in a home where love was shown by making us better and stronger. It was a home of critiquing every movement. This critique method was a language barrier and the more I tried showing "love" the harder it became for Amber. She thought I was being negative and no amount of "I Love You's" could fix the damage that was being done.

This amazing journey with Amber lasted 3 years. My journey with Amber caused me to deeply reflect on the words that came from my mouth. From the day we finally split ways I decided that "critique" was not the best method to show love.

To this day Amber and I are still dear friends and we are still connected in a deep way.

Cynthia

Where Amber was the "Spark" in my life, Cynthia was the "Calm".

It was almost ten years later when I met Cynthia. Ten years of reflection on my words and actions. But it was not ten years of peace. Peace came when Cynthia entered my life.

I remember at that time that my brother Basil and I were having a few sibling issues. Cynthia, being a peaceful person, did not like to see our pain. So she connected the both of us with a local "minister".

My meeting with this "minister" was an awakening. For the first and almost only time in my life I found myself opening up in ways I had never known existed. A simple long embraced hug from the kind woman was all it took to break down years of walls and barriers. I remember well how the flood gates of emotions emptied from my body and how the tears would not stop for hours.

To this day I do not know how this stranger affected me in such a way but it is what I needed in my life. I have forever been impacted.

My efforts to communicate and experience love came full circle when Cynthia handed me a copy of "The Five Love Languages" written by Gary Chapman.

Had I known earlier what was in those pages I may not have made so many relationship mistakes. Or at least my journey would not have been as difficult.

Today I live unencumbered and free. I take time to work on those love languages within myself and with the world around me. I am taking time to figure out who I am and I am determining what love language I need from my next partner in life.

Chapter 8
Processing

Remember our friends the frogs, who we first met sitting on a log, talking about taking an action, but never following through? Recalling a fable, let's revisit one of these frogs, now hopping around a farmyard.

This frog decided to investigate the barn. He was curious, and somewhat careless, and fell into a pail half-filled with fresh milk. He was not a big frog, and not particularly strong, and as he swam about attempting to reach the top of the pail, he found that the sides of the pail were too high to reach.

The frog tried to stretch his back legs and push off the bottom of the pail. He found it was too deep.

But this frog was determined not to give up and he continued to struggle. He kicked, and squirmed, and kicked more vigorously and squirmed harder, until finally, all his churning in the milk had turned the milk into a huge hunk of butter.

The butter was now solid enough for the frog to climb onto and get out of the pail. The frog, now wiser and stronger from his physical exertions, said "Never give up."

Throughout my life as a learner, I've often experienced the frustration of the frog at the bottom of the milk pail: pushing, and kicking, and squirming, but with seemingly little or no positive results. From a young age through today, I can focus intently, or hyper-focus, on certain activities, such as simultaneously absorbing the texts of recorded books while playing video games. But when it came to schoolwork, I had a hard time staying on task.

I've never lacked the ability to pay attention, but I've struggled with the ability to control what I pay attention to. A trained physician would recognize signs of Attention Deficit Disorder (ADD). I'm far from alone.

The Centers for Disease Control and Prevention reports that 5.4 million children ages 4-17 have been diagnosed with ADD, and those diagnoses appear to be increasing by as much as 5.5 percent annually. The CDC also reports that approximately 5 percent of children with ADD have some form of Learning Disability (LD). These challenges don't stop at childhood; adults with this diagnosis must continue to develop coping strategies to achieve at their best potential.

In the sweltering summer of 1985, I arrived in the United States with my parents, Nabil and Salwa. It had been a record-breaking cold winter in Georgia, with temperatures in Atlanta reaching as low as -8 degrees Fahrenheit, but Georgia's infamous mid-year heat and humidity marked the days of July. The month our Malouf family settled in Stone Mountain from Jordan, Coca-Cola announced the return of Coke Classic, which was actually its original formula, after New Coke proved to be a short-lived flop. The music of an emerging 21-year-old recording star, Whitney Houston, dominated local radio airwaves. I was little aware of these happenings. I just figured we would live in Georgia for a while, then return to Jordan. Our move almost felt like an extended vacation.

By late summer, I had enrolled at Rowland Elementary School in DeKalb County, near Stone Mountain. I approached my new school and classmates a quiet and withdrawn kid, an immigrant from the Middle East who spoke only Arabic. My struggles as a fourth grader soon began.

You learned of some of my early elementary school struggles in an earlier chapter. Learning English for me was like starting all over again, like I was learning to read for the first time. My first halting attempts to read were mini occasions for celebration. But then, instead of gradual progress, I continued to stumble. I'm sure that because my English was so limited, my teachers must have wondered if I simply could not master more complex skills, or perhaps they guessed I had a learning disability, such as dyslexia. "Or maybe it is Fadi's lack of focus," my teacher may have asked. "Perhaps that's what is keeping him from getting through a written page?"

I now know more about how ADD itself can also cause difficulty in reading. If ADD symptoms are not properly treated, children may find it harder to focus on learning letter sounds. Some readers with ADD may impulsively substitute a word with the same first letter as the one on the page.

Other research has suggested that children with ADD are significantly delayed in developing their internal language (the mind's voice). This private voice inside our minds is what we use to talk with ourselves, contemplate events, and direct our own behavior. If this inner voice is delayed due to ADD, it can interfere with a person's ability to read and follow directions carefully, follow through on rules and instructions, or complete plans and "to-do-lists."

When combined with their difficulties with working memory, this problem with self-talk can significantly interfere with reading comprehension, especially complex, uninteresting, or extended reading assignments. Perhaps this helps explains some of my struggles with reading.

Being pulled from class for extra support did not help. When I missed a class, even one hour of instruction, I felt as if I had missed out completely, and might never again catch up. I was sorely disappointed when later I was told I could not finish my Fourth Grade year. I would have to repeat that grade. I didn't know then that the decision might benefit me in later years.

Discovering What Works for Me

As you have discovered I've fought hard since elementary school to compensate for academic difficulties I suffered because of ADD. By the time college had come around I had spent thousands on several different types of treatments which included the brief usage of typical ADD drugs.

When you have ADD, it's easy to think that there's something wrong with you. It's okay to be different. ADD isn't an indicator of capability or intelligence. Certain things may challenge you more, but that doesn't mean you can't find your niche and achieve success. There is a long, very impressive list of people who achieved great success despite ADD, including President George Bush (both father and son), Alexander Graham Bell, Albert Einstein, Tom Cruise, Thomas Edison, the Wright Brothers, Ted Turner, Bill Gates, Jack Nicholson, Stephen Hawking, and Alfred Hitchcock. The key is to find out what your strengths are and capitalize on them.

I believe that everyone has elements of Attention Deficit Disorder in them, although only 4 percent of adults in western countries are diagnosed. I embrace the traits that I see in my friends and loved ones with ADD and, which I'm proud to say, I see in myself: incredible passion, energy, creativity, out-of-the-box thinking, and a constant flow of original ideas.

I've long ago discovered by using several techniques like the *"StrengthsFinder"* assessment what I'm good at and have worked steadily to establish an environment to support these strengths. All of my life, I've felt tremendous gratitude to people I feel are better than me, who can make me a better person. Often these have been people older than me, who have more life experience and the wisdom that comes from living. I surround myself with these people. They teach me much and make me stronger.

Among the lessons I've learned about myself – helpful ways in which I can control impulsivity and disorganization -- is to bring together people with multiple talents. I handle all tasks I'm best equipped to manage, and seek out others with skill sets I lack. In recent months, I've been fortunate to assemble a team of gifted individuals, all of whom bring specific talents and ideas which complement one another. We are bringing our shared dreams to fruition.

Building a trusted support system of people who can fill in your areas of weakness as you use your strengths to help them reach their own potential -- is one of the most important things you can do. As you commit to sharing yourself to help others, you also need people rallying people around you to help you where you are weakest.

Experience has taught me that I work well under pressure. I take on many tasks at once. My thought processes are always moving. With multiple stimuli, I work most effectively, at my highest level. Some people claim they even can't chew gum and drive a car at the same time. That's not me.

And yet, there is a downside to having so much going on at once. Sometimes I start so many projects that I have a hard time seeing them all to completion.

That is when having a support team makes a difference. As you decide what is most important in your life, you begin to prioritize your goals, and you turn to those who can help you. You never keep your goals a secret. You announce your intentions and the results you seek, because you never know if the person listening can make a key contribution to the end result.

Determining Your Boulders

Can you identify which of your goals are most urgent to you? Have you written them down with specific dates for their completion? Many of you will answer "No." Writing down your goals, sharing those goals with others, and committing to intentional acts to reach those goals will yield results. But where do you start?

I follow a Boulders System for reaching my goals. My first awareness of such a concept originated from a tale Stephen Covey shared in *First Things First*, in which a lecturer illustrated a lesson in establishing priorities using a jar with sand and pebbles. In my mind, I liken areas of my life to an empty pond, which I am going to fill up with ideas and actions that matter to me. Once a pond is filled, that phase of my life will be complete. Beside each dugout pond I have a stack of large boulders, piles of rock of varying sizes, and mounds of dirt and sand.

My highest priorities, those matters that are most important to me, are my boulders. Since these are the goals that I most want to achieve – the items that will make the greatest difference to me and others – I first throw these into the dry pond bed. Those boulders therefore get my first attention, and I know they'll settle into the base of the pond. These boulders become the foundation. I also think of a friend, who begins to fill his pond by shoveling in the sand and dirt, then trying to toss in his rocks and boulders. But my friend's pond quickly fills up, and most of his boulders are left out.

Learning this valuable lesson, I make sure all my boulders are pushed in first. Then I shovel in the smaller rocks, which represent my second most important level of priorities. Finally, I pack in the remaining gaps and crevices with the sand, the least important items, and cover it all up with dirt that I spread over the top. Objectives met. It's time to start preparing the next pond.

It takes time to fill a pond. I have to identify the boulders before I ever push them down into the hole. It is hard work, and often I call on the help of others to move the boulders, and even the rocks. Some call it persistence, or having an iron will, but rarely do goals get reached without sweat equity and sacrifice.

Few things are as frustrating as doing the work and not seeing the desired results. But even as the frog trapped in the milk pail discovered, being persistent and mixing up his techniques eventually yielded him the result he desired.

There is one more important lesson from the frog who turned milk into butter. He never lost his focus on his goal and objectives. No matter what it took, he was determined to get out of that pail. Had he lost focus, he might never have escaped that pail of milk.

Focus and motivation are a challenge, but doing a little bit very well, consistently over time, will help you stay motivated. Identify your boulders, and take care of the important issues first.

Chapter 9
Light In The Dark

Salwa Malouf became nearly speechless in 1989 when her husband Nabil presented her with an unforgettable birthday gift – a new Ford Mercury Cougar. The 1989 Cougar, with a supercharged V6 engine and automatic gearbox, embodied the agility and elegance of a mountain lion. Salwa's new silver coupe, sporting European lines and sport bucket seats, featured a modern interior with performance-minded analog gauges. Its carriage rested on a fully independent rear suspension, allowing each wheel on the same axle to react to a bump in the road independently of each other. Motor Trend Magazine recognized the Cougar as its Runner-Up for "Car of the Year." It was truly a gift of love from my father Nabil to his beloved wife.

By May 1993, my father was ready to pay off Salwa's Cougar. He called the bank where he financed the car loan to confirm the pay-off balance, unaware of complications involving insurance. Nabil, who had consistently maintained full comprehensive, collision and liability insurance, was shocked to learn that the lienholder claimed he owed $6,000 more than he believed he owed on the car.

Due to possible internal confusion, the bank had tacked on three years' of collision and comprehensive insurance premiums to Nabil's car loan, and had charged him for the additional insurance without his knowledge. Learning of this error during his phone inquiry, Nabil delayed the payoff for a few months, until he could resolve the issue with the bank. By late August, with less than a year of payments remaining, Nabil had an appointment with his banker to pay off the Cougar.

On Wednesday night, August 25, Nabil Malouf heard a noise outside his house. He confronted a subcontracted tow truck crew, men who had arrived at his Stone Mountain home to try to remove his wife's Mercury Cougar from his garage. Police arrived a few minutes later and ordered the wrecker crew to leave, stating that they had no business on Nabil's private property.

The next morning, August 26, Nabil drove the Cougar to his workplace, an exporter of heavy equipment parts, about 12 miles from home. He had an appointment that morning to pay off the car, but planned to work until the bank opened. He would settle the issue and return the car to his wife before returning to work. "Don't worry, there is a mistake," he had told Salwa.

Five minutes after Nabil entered his office, his secretary told him someone was trying to tow his car away. The tow truck from the night before had either followed him to work or was waiting for him nearby.

Nabil rushed outside, confronting the assistant driver, who already had hooked up the Cougar to the tow truck. Witnesses said the driver tried to hold him back. Nabil Malouf told the driver to stop, and reached for the passenger door of the truck. He tried to climb in as one of the drivers pushed him away. He tried to climb on the truck again, but slipped and fell to the ground.

One witness reported that a helper "was standing beside the tow truck telling the driver to "go, go, go" even as [Nabil Malouf] was falling under the wheel."

The right rear wheel crushed 58-year-old Nabil Malouf's chest. He died at a local hospital.

In the state of Georgia, a company cannot repossess if there is any form of breach of peace. That is defined as anything from fighting to simply saying, "Don't take my car." Our family sued for actual and punitive damages and agreed to a seven-figure settlement. Legal fees consumed much of the money.

My brother Baseem, oldest son of Nabil and Salwa, recovered the car by writing a check. Salwa, overcome with grief at the loss of her husband, drove the silver Cougar he died to protect for her until its transmission failed.

The death of my father, in such an unexpected and violent way, came as a crushing blow. I was 17-years-old the day my father died, and was wholly unprepared to lose him. I still needed to spend time with my dad, to do things with him. Such shared experiences had created a space for me to open up and talk.

My father was authentic. He could be a calming force and a reliable source of guidance when I needed advice. The void created by my father's tragic death would be impossible to fill.

Nabil had taught his sons about true masculinity. As I matured, I learned through my father that manliness means strong character, quiet strength, self-control, and soldiering through adversity without whining. Nabil exhibited an internal toughness, not complaining, but not letting others tell him what to do.

With my father's passing, I realized I would become the man of the house. My older brothers had already reached adulthood. I would have to think about things I had never before considered. I would need to keep things under control.

I took to heart the words of my brother Basil, who forewarned me that my life would never be the same.

"You're not 17 anymore. You're now 27," Basil told me after our father died. "You've got to take responsibility."

Sometimes feelings of anger surfaced; anger at being robbed of the most significant man in my life. Gone was the mentor who could help me and validate me as I abandoned childhood for adulthood.

A direct connection to my identity had vanished. Nabil Malouf was with me since the beginning, the root back to my ancestors, both biologically and psychosocially. His paternal lessons were powerful. It was Nabil who had taught me to keep my head up, to look beyond my challenges, and to focus on where I want to be.

I would know love from others as I came to terms with my father's passing. In time I would learn to express my love in words as well as deeds. But no one could ever love me with the unique feeling of attachment that my father gave. It is an intense and unique love that only a father can give. I would grieve at that loss.

In honor of my father, I cultivated the strength to move forward, to improve myself, and make my life count. I realized over time that my father would never really leave me.

I learned that when you love someone, they become a part of you. They are always with you, even after they die.

Chapter 10
Strong At The Core

It may surprise my friends to read that I consider myself a private person. As I built my career as a fitness trainer, and later gained notice as an entrepreneur and personal development expert, I began to look at myself from the inside out. I questioned my motivations in hopes of discovering my truest passion, the driving force behind my ambitions. We all need to have such self-introspection, but for some people, inflated ego or simple pride masks their true intentions.

What drives me is not a desire for fame. While approval from others for a job well done is a basic affirmation we all appreciate, that's never been the fuel behind my fire. Even at age 21, when I had already appeared in a profile entitled "Human Nature" in *Sports and Fitness Magazine*, followed by several years of Top 3 finishes in international bodybuilding competition, I never sought the spotlight. In nine years as a bodybuilding champion, I never commissioned photographs or staged publicity campaigns. Promoting myself wasn't my aim. Perhaps I lacked the confidence?

I've never sought to be famous, or put myself out before the public to draw attention to myself, for my own glory or enrichment. Offers came to me anyway, and I was fortunate to appear in several magazines, performed in TV commercials, and had supporting roles in motion pictures. As a physical fitness trainer, I've personally conducted more than 64,000 training sessions for clients of all walks of life. Seeing my clients' transformations is incredibly gratifying.

Still, I inwardly reflected as to what truly matters to me. I sought to discover what most ignited my passions. Recalling the Comfort Challenge concept shared by Tim Ferriss in *The 4-hour Work Week,* I pondered a *Reflective Action,* an introspective question that helps me focus my thoughts: *How do I best use my time? When am I at my strongest?*

I didn't discover the answers overnight. I decided to develop a system to help me discover what truly matters most to me and then take actionable steps toward that passion. This process, which I will share in this chapter, led me to finally understand what I'm wired to do and why.

In an earlier chapter, I shared with you my personal Core Values. Your own personal Core Values, complete with actionable items, are the foundation of your self-expression, success, and happiness. I also shared with you my personal Mission Statement, and my dreams and goals. All of these values, and goals, and mission statement originated during the first of five steps, in a process I think of as the "5 Steps to Creating Life Balance."

5 Steps to Creating Life Balance

I. **Determine What is Most Important to You in Life**. This step involves six specific intentions, or intentional behaviors.

1. The first intention is to create a set of Core Values. This requires self-examination. Define what is most important to you and learn how to effectively communicate your values to others. For each value, list

Action Items, or specific tasks you can do to help you live out that Core Value.

    2. The second intention is to create a personal Mission Statement. This statement is typically one sentence, and clearly states your life mission. My Mission is "to be a man of my word, a bold leader, and an inspiration for growth and love for every family, friend, and partner."

    3. Next is to create your Dreams and goals. Write these down and visit them daily. Give specific dates to your goals.

    4. Prioritize your day. Use the Boulder System (explained in Chapter 8) to set and follow through on your daily priorities.

    5. Write down your intentions and goals. There is great power in writing down your goals and steps you'll take to meet them. It makes you accountable and serves as a resource to track your progress.

    6. Create a Reflective Action. This can be an introspective question that helps you focus your thoughts. It usually involves completing a simple task that supports your goals and Core Values. Here's an example: Send a personal note to three family members you haven't spoken to in more than one month.

II. Drop the Habits and Affirmations That Do Not Benefit Your Purpose.

    1. Document where you are spending your time and money. You will quickly recognize what you value.

    2. Drop any unnecessary activities. We can find ourselves bogged down in activities that support our Boulders and don't support our goals. These can drain us of energy and time spent pursing what really matters to us.

    3. Become aware of your quiet thoughts. Reflective

Action: Define what is most important to you and learn how to effectively communicate your values to others.

III. **Protect Your Private Time.**

1. If you don't have integrity with yourself, eventually you won't have it anywhere else.

2. Who keeps you accountable to your personal and professional growth? How is that accountability accomplished?

3. Reflective Actions: Meditate for 15 minutes three days a week. Do this for three consecutive weeks. For one day, when asked to do something extra, decline in a respectful manner. Be sure to be direct and clear. Don't fall into a trap of accepting the request after you declined.

IV. **Accept Help to Balance Your Life.**

1. "Life is a two-way road." Allow people to do things for you and develop trust in others.

2. Don't assume that your partner or the people in your life can read your mind. Understand your valued interests and express them in a clear, respectful, and loving way.

3. Reflective Action: Make a list of five to 10 items, small or large, that need to be done and request people in your life to help.

V. **Plan Fun and Relaxation.**

1. You make time for everything else. Why not this?

2. Put it on your schedule. Scheduling it makes you much more likely to plan ahead, save money, submit deposits, and build excitement for the event.

3. Exercising is relaxing and fun. Play should be an integral part of a healthy and balanced life!

4. After completing Steps 1-4 of the 5 Steps to Creating Life Balance, complete this Reflective Action: Take action on your planned goals and dreams, and play your way to success!

It takes energy, sometimes a great deal of it, to follow a plan to completion. But expending such energy is necessary most times to get something meaningful done. As most any successful and happy individual will attest, the core – the center or heart -- of one's physical being is the most important part of the human body. As you strengthen your body and sharpen your mind, your intellect and emotional, psychological and spiritual state begin to match your physical dexterity.

Getting to that point requires clearly understanding who you are and deciding where you want to be. Follow a plan for living by your Core Values to reach the goals that matter most to you, and you will start to become your possibilities!

So what did the 5 Steps to Achieving Life Balance help me to discover about myself? I want to make a positive difference in somebody else's life. I can help others define their dreams and achieve measureable and lasting results, through mastering their mind, spirit, and body. I want to help people live STRONG, by improving their lifestyles as a result of healthy living. I help people realize the results they want.

Chapter 11

Intentions

Like a trail runner exploring unfamiliar woods, I found myself unacquainted with the direction my life was taking as I entered adulthood. Often engaged in introspection following my father's death, I worked through how I could produce results that would make my life matter. I permitted myself to dream big, bolstered by my brothers' encouragement, and a force of will to endure and thrive.

Young in mind and experience, and driven hard to excel physically in the weight room, I adopted a motto: *Feel the burn and be accomplished!* I was all too familiar with personal failures, yet I chose to *honor* those failures as necessary learning experiences.

Honored by failure! Some of the most accomplished men and women in history failed numerous times before they experienced success. My *response* to failure would determine the outcome. If I began to doubt myself, I would recall words attributed to basketball legend Michael Jordan: "I've missed more than 9,000 shots in my career. I've lost almost 300 games. 26 times I've been trusted to take the game winning shot and missed. I've failed over and over and over again in my life and that is why I succeed."

My personal affirmations, those little voices within my thoughts that motivated and encouraged, could sometimes prove disempowering, if negative thoughts were allowed to slip in. Pain, I discovered, was most commonly associated with a disempowering affirmation.

It's hard, I might think as I lifted through a fourth set of barbell rows, burning under the strain as I strengthened my deltoid and back muscles. *Does doing hard things motivate me or charge me up?*

Can't get there, my mind might argue, as I powered through a superset of rope pull-downs, on my knees, waist bent forward, deeply twisting each elbow forward to the opposite thigh. Then reminding myself that the pulls would tighten my upper abdominals and obliques, I would counter, S*o what CAN you get to?*

As demands on my schedule increased, I recognized that I occasionally thought some of the same disempowering affirmations; so many others cried out: *It's too much time*, or, *I don't know if I'll get to tha*t and etc. Through self-discipline, I focused on responses that redirected me toward my goals. *What is too much or too little? How much TIME is WORTH spending towards my health? How is using the words "I don't" or "I can't" working for me? With what do I replace those negative words?*

As I discovered the power of positive affirmations and establishing goals, I began to build a career I never expected. At age 20, in response to the growing demand and public interest in health and fitness, I founded Body By Fadi, an elite personal training company. Learning on the job, I prepared and implemented a strategic marketing plan, conducted research and analysis, and over time produced annual sales exceeding six figures. I was a hands-on executive, overseeing personal training, conducting nutrition counseling sessions, and managing all aspects of my business. My clients kept me traveling, from Atlanta to Miami, and California to New York.

As I sculpted my physique and transformed into an Adonis, I welcomed the attention I received from admiring women, and I rarely lacked for dates. My inborn competitiveness and encouragement from weight lifting officials prompted me to enter international bodybuilding competitions, where shy guys finish last. I was motivated to become the world's youngest natural professional body builder.

Between 1996 and 2004, I competed in several shows a year, revealing a showman's spirit and perfect form. I never placed less than third in any competition I entered.

By my mid-20s, I had reached a crossroads. I was earning six figures, and despite a host of serious injuries, my physical abilities remained off the chart. Twice, both times playing volleyball with friends, I heard the tell-tale pop and cracking sound of a torn Anterior Cruciate Ligament (ACL), followed by sharp pain on the outside and back of my knee. I endured a lingering shoulder injury. On another occasion, while sprinting during interval training, I accelerated quickly and stretched fibers within my powerful hamstring muscle, causing the fibers to tear and bleed within the muscle.

One of my most unforgettable injuries occurred during a weight training session, when I experienced sudden wrenching pain and a tearing sensation in my chest as my pectoralis major muscle ruptured. This chest muscle, the larger of the two pectoralis muscles, works to push the arms in front of the body, such as in a bench press maneuver. Bruising soon followed. Fortunately, with time, good nutrition and rest I was eventually able to return to high-level sports and activities.

During this period of development as an athlete, I decided to try out for the Georgia Force, a professional Arena Football League team. I had the attributes that coaches love: strength, speed, and agility. I had a 43-inch vertical jump, enough gravity-busting height to easily dunk a basketball. I was strong as a bear, bench pressing 550 pounds, squatting 680 pounds and able to dead-lift 750 pounds, all with a sculpted body weight of 260. I owned three high school records in two different sports, one in track and two in weightlifting, for squats and the dead-lift.

With my growing success as a trainer and entrepreneur, I pondered my interest in Arena football. Perhaps it stemmed from my school days, to the first time I joined a football team, but broke a finger on the second day of practice and was forced to stop playing. I later made another attempt at football prior to graduation, but just as with my short-lived Arena experience, I admit I didn't really know the game.

By 2000, I reached athletic levels I could not have imagined as a skinny kid with brittle bones who was bullied and beaten by his neighbors. I was named Overall Winner of the 2000 World Nationals (SNBF) Super Natural Bodybuilding and Fitness Championships and later named Overall Winner in the 2000 International Musclemania Tour World Natural Bodybuilding Championships. My events were televised worldwide, giving me my first exposure to an international audience.

By 28 years of age, I had transformed myself into a lifetime drug-free professional bodybuilder, a fitness specialist, spokesmodel, and performance nutritional specialist. And I grew into a super-sized champion: a 6 foot-1 inch frame, harboring 245 pounds of muscle, lean and toned.

The professional accolades continued. In 2004, the last year I competed internationally as a bodybuilder, I placed second in the Team Universe Heavyweight Class and won the NPC Eastern Seaboard Super Heavyweight title. I am widely regarded by national fitness magazines and numerous professional associations as having one of the world's most symmetrical and defined natural physiques.

I had faced my giants, and as I did I gained mastery over my mindset, my nutrition, and my muscles. So effectively had I, as a natural professional bodybuilder, learned to maximize the speed of my metabolism, I was able to maintain 6.2 percent body fat year-round, with hardly any cardiovascular exercise.

As magazine editors and producers called on me for photo shoots, film scenes, or commercials, I occasionally built some cardio into my training, typically a week or two before the filming or photo session. My goal was simply to shed some water retention. Acting lessons with mentors helped me improve my camera presence.

My specialty, years in development and skillfully honed to perfection, was understanding how to maximize lean muscle to increase metabolism and burn away fat. I had become a fat burning machine, working non-stop, 24 hours a day, 7 days a week. I understood the key role of balanced nutrition and its relationship to the needs of the human body and its 640 muscles. I was more eager than ever to help others transform their own bodies with the knowledge I had gained.

I had redefined my professional focus. My goal would be to help others muster the courage and strength to make the conscience efforts necessary to reinvent their fitness and produce new results for their lives. I would show them how.

Chapter 12
Investment

I am the culmination of all the people who have influenced me in the past 38 years. Much of who I am today is the result of my life experiences and the relationships I've built. I've had little or no control over some of what I experienced, but many things I've lived through are directly related to choices I made.

I guess that's true of all of us. We're born where we're born, into the families God gives us, and we figure out a way to carry on through life. Until we become adults, we have little say over where we live, or with whom. There is little doubt that the people who surround us as we grow up have great influence on our views and our perspectives on how things are, or should be.

The role models in my life have shaped me in unknown ways. My father Nabil deeply loved my mother Salwa. Together they brought a daughter and three sons into the world. My sister Rhonda is the elder, Baseem and Basil come next and I am the youngest of the group.

Each of us has slightly different personalities which sometimes made for conflict. As the youngest sibling, I learned not only from my own mistakes, but from my siblings as well.

My father, who died when I was 17, was authoritative. His word was final, but he was also patient and calm. The appropriate response to his directives was

"Yes, Sir," followed immediately by the action he wished us to take.

Nabil, which means *Nobel*, worked hard for his family, and he was a dependable provider. He impacted his workplace, a company that exported heavy equipment parts, but consistently managed to make it home for dinner with his family. He enjoyed a nightly glass of Scotch or sipped on another favorite whiskey, Jack Daniels Black Label.

Growing up, of course, I had no idea I would lose my father before I graduated from high school. His passing at age 58 makes my memories of time spent with him even more precious. They provide snapshots into his personality.

I've never been a smoker, but in Jordan, the spring before we moved to Georgia, some fellow 8-year-olds convinced me I should try cigarettes, a fact which they all had hid from their older brothers. My father got word of it. One evening, very coolly, he handed me a pack of Benson & Hedges 100s, and calmly announced, "Go ahead, Fadi, and smoke it."

I gave him an inquisitive look, and glanced down at the pack of cigarettes, and looked at him again. He just waited. I opened the silver package, pulled out a smoke, and he lit it with a match. A couple of puffs later I was through with smoking for the rest of my life.

I remember riding in a jeep with my father, and sharing beefy jerky, and meals of chicken wings, one of our favorites. I also recall a night on I-285, the Atlanta perimeter, when he allowed me to drive. He fell asleep in the passenger seat, and I kept missing the exit and driving around and around the by-pass. I was only 13 years old.

"When we get home," he said after I finally found the exit, "tell you mother how many cars we passed."

In my family, service was the language of love. That was particularly true of my mother, who didn't believe in expressing love through words and terms of endearment.

During our childhood, if Mom cleaned you, and cooked your dinner, she did her job. She modeled a lifestyle of service, and that was what she expected of us.

After we moved to the United States, my mother came to feel that American youth were much too liberated. She would not let that happen to me. Expressing my emotions, and outwardly sharing feelings of affection, were things I could not do.

My sister Randa, who joined us in Stone Mountain in the mid-1980s after she left an abusive marriage in Saudi Arabia, treated me with the maternal affection I craved. She would comfort me, rub my hair, or hold me when I felt sad. To this day I'm not sure why she was so different from the rest of my family.

When I was younger, and my family traveled extensively, Rhonda first assumed the role of my mother. She practically raised me at times, and in my youthful eyes, I sometimes viewed her more like a mother to me than my own. This confused me, and it somehow didn't feel right. It was like I had two, but very different mothers.

I dearly love my mother Salwa. But growing up, I was unable to channel that love towards her, because she was authoritative and traditional, what today we might call "old school." My mother is a powerful individual, who fed me, cared for me, and provided for me in many necessary ways, but she was madly in love with my father. Her love for my father was paramount. My sister Rhonda, 17 years older, understood this and filled in emotionally where gaps existed for me.

I've since shared with Rhonda my early feelings, how as a child I viewed her as my primary caretaker, a beloved maternal presence, but with guilt. Essentially, I thought the love that I felt for my sister was the kind of love I was only supposed to feel for my mother.

"I loved you so much, like a mother figure," I explained to my sister. "But I felt ashamed for loving you, even though I know you loved and cared about me."

Childhood memories with Baseem, 12 years my senior, are pleasant, but brief. A quiet man with a gentle spirit, he has a wry sense of humor I've always appreciated. I recall small experiences with him, such as taking photos of lightning, a boat ride, a scuba dive, or playing on the beach. Sometimes his youthful mistakes taught me valuable lessons, too, such as when he disregarded a curfew, or sneaked out of our house during the middle of the night. I observed his consequences for such disobedience, solemnly vowing not to subject myself to similar anguish.

I've shared much deeper experiences with my brother Basil, who assumed a role as my father while I lived with him some as I worked towards independence. I credit him with pushing me, always challenging me to work harder.

Basil is a very practical man, who believes in work, work, and more work. Sometimes his intensity, and his constant urgency, falls into the extremes.

As I was developing into a world class bodybuilder, he trained me like a military drill sergeant, motivating me with stick and guilt – good cop, bad cop. During these trainings, he inflicted pain on me, some good and some bad. Mostly good, I guess.

I remember as a kid, when Basil would keep me while my parents were out, I might get slapped by a banana, just because. I used to feel animosity toward him, but now I realize his aggression was just his way of motivating me to act.

After learning of our father's death, Basil didn't give me much time for bereavement. He made it clear that my time had come to grow up. That was a heavy challenge to hang on a grieving teenager.

Mentors

That autumn of 1993 I began a career as a personal trainer, while still in high school. I soon met Paul Coleman, a hulking man, originally from Buffalo, New York, whose charisma and talent in the gym inspired me to become better and stronger. Basil was first to place me on an intense weight training program and Paul's background in exercise science and nutrition proved invaluable to my development.

I managed to graduate from Brookwood High and later entered business school in nearby Lawrenceville, struggling mightily as I divided my time between core classes and three different jobs. I had no choice but to grow up. Constantly at work, living off tap water and cheap canned tuna, and juggling coursework at Gwinnett Technical College, I felt the cold dousing of harsh reality. In the darkest times, when I knew I had to pull through, I reminded myself that it's easy to quit but hard to live with it afterward. I chased away whispers of negative self-talk:

"You're not good enough, strong enough, smart enough." Instead, I prepared to battle for my dreams.

I can reflect now with fondness, but during those years of struggle I felt a bit like Scotsman William Wallace, mired in a desperate and fierce fight for survival, as depicted in Mel Gibson's movie *Braveheart*. Indeed, trying to finish college, still deficient in literacy skills, while hammering out a career, proved to be a fight to the finish. But I expected to succeed. I knew that it was *my* responsibility to make my dreams a reality. Much happened as a result, often unexpected, but I have never regretted the journey I took.

I treasure the experiences I've shared with my family and my mentors. Memories fade, and details become blurred, but in recollection, all the time we spent together is priceless. Recalling the stories passed forward, the hard-earned wisdom shared, and numerous sacrifices made, I'm flushed with gratitude. As Les Brown observed, "Someone's sitting in the shade today because someone planted a tree a long time ago."

Time together with my family gave me opportunities to make changes within myself that empowered me to be a better human being. I've sought out forgiveness for wrongs I've incurred, and sought to forgive.

Shared experiences changed how we now see each other and how we view ourselves.

I'll never again get to share a laugh with my father as we split an order of chicken wings, or enjoy an inspiring workout with Paul Coleman, who passed away in 2010. But great men like these, and other, men and women who are still in my life, remind me of the importance of helping others, of sharing wisdom, or a compliment, or even a tangible gift of some sort while you can. Life is short and we should not wait to share our gifts and talents, and for most of all, our time.

Chapter 13

Ten Percent Stronger

You want to do more than just survive in this world. You want to excel in it. And you should indeed seek to excel in it, to contribute to it, and to give something back upon receipt. Most importantly, you should be the first to give with no need for return.

In doing so, you secure your life's path and journey. You affirm, acknowledge and embrace. Others will be inspired to live the same way. You shine your light on your fellow human beings, and they are illuminated.

The Ten Percent Stronger Principle means you commit to give 10 percent of your time to help others, and invest 10 percent of your money for causes that improve people's lives. You commit to improve your own health, and your economic well-being, with an ongoing goal to bless others and make the world a better place.

By living Ten Percent Stronger, there is no me or you. There is only *us*. Self-centeredness will fall away, replaced by production, profit, and increase in every aspect of your life. Unproductive and unhealthy actions that failed you in the past will begin to succeed in the present, as you move to secure a better future for all of us.

It all begins with the Ten Percent Stronger Principle. Your life lived Ten Percent Stronger is really lived at 100 percent and to the umpteenth degree. You pay your blessings forward, establish seed money for projects, concentrate on the good in others, and accentuate the positive. When you focus on the positive, things get better, just as when you focus on negativity things get worse.

Anyone can make an impact. You don't need to be wealthy to begin. Earning $200.00 and investing $20.00 (10 percent) adds up over time. As you employ the principle of Ten Percent Stronger, you invest in all of our lives. You'll see gains in your own savings and Individual Retirement Accounts, but that's not your motivation. The return to you is ten-fold, as you acknowledge your gratitude to others and pay kindness forward.

Somehow, that's the way it works. But you don't have to concern yourself with the details.

All you have to do is focus on the intentions behind your actions. In this way, there is no choice between you, your money, and your life. Your money ends up working for you and, importantly, for others in your life. You will begin to reap the rewards of unselfishness, and ultimately realize unending and increasingly greater success.

You will become a positive human being. You begin to comprehend what it means to send out good vibrations with sincere intentions. These positive vibrations reflect back to you in the form of a growing bank account, and the clear and positive accounting of your life. You secure your place in the lives of others.

Living the Ten Percent Stronger Principle does not only secure your economic status. That's just a fringe benefit. Your core ideal and objective is to share, to become generous (to generate), and to encourage (to give courage). You can apply these objectives to every aspect of your life, beyond your economic status. Yet, a sound economic status frees you from the worries of the world and allows you to more easily concentrate on helping others.

We all know the old adage, "Which comes first – the chicken or the egg?" The answer is both. Nothing is singular and no action stands alone. One action ignites another. Your commitment to your health and fitness will make you work more effectively in the other areas of your life.

By adopting the Ten Percent Stronger Principle, you *take* action. You become the chicken and the egg as a metamorphosis takes place. You cross the road to get to a better place and mark the way for your peers, friends, co-workers, children, and your family. At your core you become part of all of our families, by way of living Ten Percent Stronger.

With the Ten Percent Stronger Principle, you wipe away fear, uneasiness, and greed. You begin to recognize our common humanity. We all arrive in this world completely dependent on the kindness of others. We grow up and learn behaviors that help us cope. Some of our learned behaviors hold us back.

A life committed to giving and sharing with others helps you relearn how life was supposed to be lived before you acquired habits and behaviors that often failed. Any "No Percent Questions" you once struggled with become irrelevant when you follow the Ten Percent Stronger Principle.

For the principle to work, you must ignore differences in people and start concentrating on that which makes us the same. We all have the same basic needs, none the least of which is to be unconditionally loved. And by living Ten Percent Stronger, you set no conditions, only purity in action. That purity is in the execution of your intentions and the results of those actions, which are multiplied by the pure actions of others.

In time you learn to share. You share your knowledge, your wisdom, your heart, your smile, and most importantly, your time – which, by way of the joyful memories you'll leave behind, becomes infinite.

In this way, life at Ten Percent Stronger teaches you that your time, more than anything, is the most you can offer anyone. You can invest time with a friend who may be suffering from low self-esteem. You can spend time with a family member who is experiencing a serious illness. You can share time with a friend who may simply be lonely. Those with whom you invest your time will give back to you.

And it only takes a *ten percent* of your time. That's living Ten Percent Stronger. Live stronger that way and you'll deliver strength to others.

Chapter 14
B.A.L.A.N.C.E

    We live in a country where more than two-thirds of the population is overweight or obese. Look around and you see it everywhere. Nearly half of Americans surveyed in 2011 said they'd like restaurants to offer healthier items with fewer fats and calories, but only 23 percent tend to order those foods. (Associated Press) As a society, we are out of balance.

    The imbalance spans across the generations. Today's kids are entering into adulthood 20 pounds heavier than in 1960. By the time children are 4 to 5 years old, 60 percent of them have lost their ability to self-regulate food intake. Men and women in their middle-age years naturally experience a slowdown of their metabolism, the process their body performs to burn and use calories. This slowing of our metabolism makes it even more important for people 40 years and over to exercise regularly and to lower their calorie intake to prevent weight gain. Simply put, unless a 47-year-old is exercising regularly to burn calories, many of the calories he or she consumes daily will convert into even more pounds and unwanted weight gain. Keep in mind that this is also true for people of all ages. It happens every day and it is preventable.

    Creating Balance is about living a life in which you meet your needs with healthy foods and staying committed to being active. Exercising most days of the week will burn more calories, making you feel great and inspiring you to become even more active.

The standard supermarket diet is rich in sugar, saturated fat, and sodium. Salt, sugar and fats stimulate us to eat more than we need. That's why it matters that you choose foods rich in fiber, like fruits, vegetables, and whole grains. It's necessary to drink a lot of water, and choose low-fat or fat-free products, limiting those found in the dairy section. The meats you choose should be lean, like chicken, fish, or turkey without skin. Those foods are available, but you've got to choose them.

Think about the meaning of the word *Balance,* defined as a "harmonious or satisfying arrangement or proportion of parts or elements, as in a design." When your life is in Balance, you enjoy it more, and feel more in control, living with a greater sense of peace. I prefer to think of B.A.L.A.N.C.E. as an acronym, created from the first letters in a series of words that remind us how to achieve harmonious balance in our lives. B.A.L.A.N.C.E. is a foundation for My Fitness Solution Academy, a three phase fitness program I founded to help individuals achieve the healthy balanced body and lifestyle of their dreams.

Creating B.A.L.A.N.C.E. in Your Life
This amazing protocol was in large part created by: Atlanta based, Your Day ETC, spa and wellness clinic.

BREATHE: B represents the word ***Breathe***. It is essential when you are investing in your health to remember the importance of cardiovascular exercise and deep breathing to your overall health. Deep breathing increases the body's ability to process oxygen at the cellular level. Take a deep breath right now and you will feel better immediately.

AGUA: A represents the Spanish word for water, **Aqua**. It is imperative when you are pursuing fitness goals to remember to hydrate your body. The amount of water in ounces you consume daily should be equal to half your body weight, and even more when active.

LENGTHEN: L is for **Lengthening**. Stretching is an essential part of resistance training and general health. The purpose of stretching, yoga, or even chiropractic work is to avoid impingement, keep your body aligned, and increase blood flow throughout your body.

ANAEROBIC: A stands for **Anaerobic**. Strength training must be a core part of improving your body. The purpose of training with weights is to strengthen your muscles, ligaments, tendons, and bones. Resistance training also increases your metabolism, which is a key to burning fat.

NUTRITION: N is for **Nutrition**. Nutrition, the food you eat, and the vitamins you take to supplement your diet, is 80 percent of your overall healthy lifestyle. You cannot get the results that you are going for without proper nutrition. This means following the best practices for nutrition and learning new information to fuel your body. Proper nutrition and supplementation regulates metabolism, provides your sources of energy, strengthens your immune system, and facilitates recuperation.

CLEANSING: C represents the necessary act of **Cleansing**. Cleansing is a part of fitness, too. Cleansing is necessary both physically and mentally. This means cleansing your mind of those thoughts that are negative and get in the way of being successful. On the physical side, it is important to monitor your body's functions. Fasting rests the digestive system and allows for cleansing and detoxification of the body. Even the fast between your last meal of the day and the next morning's breakfast benefits your body systems. Become aware of your basic digestive patterns, such as having a regular bowel movement each day. Consider having a colonic cleansing from a qualified professional. Cleansing rids the body of toxins and toxic wastes.

ENERGIZE: E is for *Energize*. You must be mindful that you have taken steps necessary to have the energy you need to accomplish all the goals you have set for yourself. In order to do this, you must sleep well each night (8 hours recommended) and, when possible, take a 20-minute nap during the day. Meditation, massage, reading, and affirming also help increase your mental awareness and strengthen your mind. Surround yourself with those whom are like-minded and support you. Share your goals with others so that they can become part of your support network.

Creating B.A.L.A.N.C.E. in your life goes hand in hand with defining your health goals, knowing your Core Values, and determining your boulders, those priorities that should be handled above all others. When you are mindful of B.A.L.A.N.C.E . you create a quality life, which leads you to be strong and productive. Health becomes your priority. You know what results matter most to you and you have proven guidelines to lead you there.

Chapter 15
Dream-Play-Be

Dream

Wherever I go, locally or when I travel, I'm often asked, "I want to get myself fit and active again, but how do I begin?" I sometimes recognize defeat in the eyes of those who ask, but I also see sparks, that determined look of people who are finally ready to transform themselves for the better.

To all, my answer is the same. "Begin your journey with a dream! Your optimal fitness and mental well-being begins with a dream."

Olympic champions, professional athletes, supermoms and highly successful individuals use visualization techniques as their key to goal attainment. So do many "regular folks" who aren't in the public eye. As you define your dream you can plan your roadmap to success.

I tell those ready for change that developing a positive mental attitude, a desire to move forward despite the challenges, helps you unleash your unlimited potential. I often think back to my childhood, the day I struggled through fear and pain to ride a bicycle. On that rock-strewn road outside my family home, dirty and streaked in sweat, my father taught me a lesson I've held onto.

"Head up. Don't focus on the bigger rocks," he

instructed. "Concentrate on where you want to be."

He was right. Each time I thought about the rocks, or when I looked down at them, I ran over them, wobbling wildly and crashing to the ground. They were everywhere. But when I kept my head up, and focused on where I was going, I forgot about rocks. I could ride like the wind.

I had dreamed of riding my bike, just as I had once witnessed my brothers riding effortlessly on their own. I didn't fear to try, but I could not have succeeded without my father's guidance and a painful lesson in focus.

Now when I dream, I dare to fail. But without my dreams, I may never have tried, and I most certainly would not have succeeded.

Play

So what becomes of our dreams? Do they all entangle us in struggle, forcing us out of our comfort zones to writhe and twist until we finally break through? Of course not! When you engage in personal development, you should choose those activities that make life fun and exciting. With every step you take in reaching optimum fitness, affirm your gratitude for your blessings. Sharpen your forward-thinking skills by focusing on the outcomes you desire, instead of the things you don't want. If your status quo is unacceptable, decide what needs changing, and be the agent for that change.

There are many ways to play. Never is play deemed frivolous or a waste of your time. Think of your *playtime* as opportunities to align your core values with your infinite intelligence, to conquer lingering fears, and increase harmony in all your relationships.

There are at least six ways to play. Not all will fit into every day, of course, but all should become part of your lifestyle.

Six Ways to Play As You Better Yourself

1. **Contribute**: Go the extra mile by rendering some sort of service to your community, your spouse, or your family without expecting any kind of reward for it. This might be as simple as offering to walk your neighbor's dog one afternoon a week, when you know your neighbor has been extra busy taking night classes for graduate school. The walk will be good for you and the dog and your neighbor.

2. **Educate:** Read, listen to recorded books, or study printed and web-based articles for self-improvement. Business expert Brian Tracy suggests reading an hour per day in your chosen field. "This works out to about one book per week, 50 books per year, and will guarantee your success," writes Tracy.

3. **Connect:** Contact members of your "mastermind alliance" and or close personal friends. Connect with those whose guidance or opinions you value and trust, and whose areas of strength can counter your weaknesses.

4. **Physical Exercise**: Devote one hour to anything strenuous and *sometimes* fun! Cardio play can be an old-fashioned game of dodgeball or a unique obstacle course. Do some stretches and

calisthenics, then take a 20 minute run and work up a sweat. You'll get your heart rate up and burn calories! Other necessary types of physical exercise include strength training or body sculpting, speed and agility exercises, cycling, swimming, Yoga, or Pilates. Identify a 5 Kilometer race a month away, and train for it in the gym and on the trails. By race day, you'll be excited and stronger for having trained and met your goal.

5   **Recreation**: Devote time to recreational activities you enjoy. Mix it up and choose something different each time. These can include fun hobbies, like tending a garden or building birdhouses, traveling to a park and exploring the outdoors, engaging in sports or games like jump rope, badminton, or croquet, or hiking up a favorite or new trail.

6.   **Relaxation:** Practice relaxation techniques. These include meditation exercises, progressive relaxation, deep breathing, guided imagery, toe tensing, and quiet ears, an ancient Eastern meditation and an effective way to fall asleep. The University of Maryland Medical Center website (http://www.umm.edu/sleep/relax_tech.htm) offers an excellent description of several of these relaxation techniques. Just try some and be amazed at how they can help you get a good night's sleep!

BE

Once your dream is a reality, continued activity and training help you support the positive changes in your life. As you live your life transformed, you enjoy renewed energy, vitality, and appreciate your physical body. You are equipped and empowered to act with purpose and a plan to attract opportunities and success. Health and fitness are a by-product. As your general health and strength improves, you become more mentally alert, productive, and attuned to new ideas. You are eager to embrace life and Be Your Possibilities!

Chapter 16
Celebrate All Wins

      I strongly believe that life is best lived as a celebration. Every morning that you wake up, and can stand and stretch, and draw in the deep breath of a new day, is cause for celebration. When you return the smile of a child, or embrace a loved one in hugs, or rub the belly of a beloved pet nestled at your feet, you have reason to celebrate

      You can fill in your own blanks of reasons you celebrate: the rush of joy you feel after an inspired workout, fatigued, perhaps a bit sore, but satisfied; achieving a personal best finish time in a local 5 Kilometer race, knowing the run also helped raise money for a deserving cause; that magical moment you drift off into sleep, wrapped in a soft blanket, as the book you're enjoying falls open in your lap, or treating your best friend to a cup of coffee, after discovering a $20 bill under your car seat when you thought you were broke. Celebrations come in all shapes and sizes, and in all forms of disguises. No blessing is too small to overlook.

      When you decide you are tired of living your life half-healthy, or you've had enough of aching joints and blood pressure readings that keep inching up, you are positioning yourself for a win. When you trade fried potato chips for fresh baby spinach, you are creating an environment for another win. When you make the conscience decision to make your health, *your* fitness, a priority in your life, you will begin to celebrate more wins than you ever thought possible.

Each week at My Fitness Solution near Atlanta, people from all walks of life gather in a gym, or occasionally on a grassy field, intent on becoming a little stronger, or a little leaner, or a little toner. These people quickly become friends, focused not solely on their own results, but on seeing positive results in each other. Each individual soon embraces the concept of *Legion*, a mindset of being part of one group with common health goals, who work together, offer support, and celebrate *all* wins, large and small.

True, each person has his or her own place on the fitness continuum. Some want to lose 100 pounds, or 10 pounds. Others focus on burning inches off their waists. Some are sculpting their already toned bodies, for upcoming competitions or to perform better in sports. Still others, on the verge of diabetes, or suffering hypertension, or soaring cholesterol, are fighting for their lives, knowing they owe it to themselves, and their families, to rediscover the joy of eating well, being active, and living fit. Bound by poor nutrition habits, or a docile lifestyle, these people are now ready to regain control and transform to realize a life without limits. They embrace the truth in their motto,

"Nothing tastes as good as being healthy feels."

You don't have to settle. Perhaps you suffer from health complications resulting from years of weight gain or obesity. You might avoid the beach or neighborhood pool each summer because you feel shame at how you see yourself in a swimsuit. Maybe you avoid taking stairs because you're embarrassed at how hard you breathe when you reach the top. You might think yet another bowl of ice cream is the cure-all for stress, or depression, or the common cold. You deprive yourself of travel because you just get too tired. Your kids, or grandkids, want to play with you, but you simply don't have the energy.

So, you tell yourself, *this is how it is. I'll never drop this weight. I've crossed the Rubicon. I'm trapped in that no man's land – the place of no return. I'll make the best of where I am, but this is my destiny. So make room on the couch, and bring me another piece of pie, please.*

If this is how you are living, I want you to know that it is never too late to retool your life. You have to change how you think. The fact is that within you is great strength. You've always had it. When you decide to use your strength, which is more powerful than you ever imagined, you will discover how wonderful your life without limits can be!

Become the New Fit – healthy in body, clear in thought, vital and active, able to have fun and realize your dreams -- by establishing your Core Values, identifying your Boulders, redirecting your focus from your short-lived challenges to your long-term goals, while maintaining B.A.L.A.N.C.E. in your everyday lifestyle. That's Strong. That's the New Fit. That can be You.

Discussion Questions
For
STRONG *The New Fit*

Introduction
What is a "Rubicon" that you have had to cross?

Chapter 1 - *Head Up*

What is a significant lesson you learned early in life? How did that lesson influence your future decisions?

In what direction do you want your life to go?

What roadblocks keep you from reaching your goals?

Where is your focus?

Where should your focus be?

Chapter 2 - *Moving Forward*

How is your body and mind helping you in your career currently?

What is the hardest hit you've ever taken in life so far?

Chapter 3 – *Adaptations*

How is where you live now different than where you lived as a child?

How is your nutrition different?
What did you play as a child?

Did you have confidence as a child? Who encouraged you?
Who discouraged you?

What do you tell yourself daily? What is your mantra?

<u>Chapter 4 - *Persistence*</u>

What have you decided to do?

Have you jumped or are you still sitting on the log?

How do you react to challenges?

What are your life's roles?

What is your life purpose? Has it changed? Why?

What are your core values? Action items?

Whom can you trust to be honestly accountable?

What do you dream about?

<u>Chapter 5 - *Becoming*</u>

Do you remember when you stood up for yourself?

With what peripheral issues do you deal?

Do you know how to get nutrition to help your body?

How can you get this nutritional knowledge?

Chapter 6 - *Discoveries*

What do you really eat?

Keep a jot list of every food that goes into your mouth for a week.

Chapter 7 - *Finding Love*

How did you feel when you experienced a broken heart during a relationship?

What lessons did you learn from the experience?

Chapter 8 - *Processing*

What are your strengths? Weaknesses?

Do you feel you have inadequacies from your childhood that puts you at a disadvantage?

Who can you enlist to help you in an area of weakness?

How can you share your strengths with someone?

Who is your support team?

Chapter 9 - *Light in the Dark*

Have you had to move forward after a tragedy?

What people have influenced you, although you have been separated by time, death, or other reasons?

Chapter 10 - *Strong At The Core*

What is most important to you in your life?

What personal affirmations are most inspiring to you?

What are ways that you can protect your private time?

Describe a time you allowed others to do something to help you. What was the end result?

What is your Reflective Action?

Chapter 11 - *Intentions*

What failures have you honored?

What physical problems keep you from developing your strength?

Chapter 12 - *Investment*

As you grew up, how did you relate to each member of your family?

Who was a mentor?

What shared experiences influenced you?

Have you forgiven family and friends and moved on?

If life is short, who do you need to forgive?

Chapter 13 - *Ten Percent Stronger*

What action can you take immediately to begin to live your life 10 percent stronger?

Who can you help cross the road?

Who is one person to whom you can give 10 percent more time?

Chapter 14 - *B.A.L.A.N.C.E.*

After reading about BALANCE, what areas of your life are well within balance?

What areas are out of balance?

What immediate actions can you do to get an area into balance?

Chapter 15 - *Dream – Play – Be*

What are your dreams?

How can you begin playing with your dream?

With whom do you share your goals?

Who is your support?

To whom could you be accountable for your dreams?

Who gets in the way of meeting your goals?

How can you negotiate this?

How do you dream of yourself being physically fit?

What action item do you need to take to make your dream a reality?

How can you add play to your life?

Chapter 16 - *Celebrate All Wins!*

Describe wins you've experienced in the past month that give you cause to celebrate.

Have you ever accepted a life situation for what it is (such as being overweight, or having high blood pressure), instead of acting on a desire to change?

How did settling for something less than desired feel?

Do you feel that you have reached your greatest potential in most areas of your life?

What areas of your life can you improve?

Describe actions you have taken to better your life that have worked for you.

BONUS
How To Be Successful In Life

Be Extraordinary!

Be A Visionary – Decide to make the change you are looking for, establish your mission and vision statements to guide your life, learn to dream again, become the "boss" or entrepreneur of your life and take control of every decision and establish the goals to match your vision and lastly establish a vision board!

Be Prepared – Hydrate, Nourish, and Rest. Prepare for each day by getting enough sleep, hydrating properly, and fueling for performance. Create meal plans, cook your food ahead of time, create shopping list and stick to the list when you go to the grocery store. Create your workout plans ahead of time.

Use Tools – In order to build a house you need tools. And the best way to build a new body is by using a few good tools like, our online Virtual Trainer for your workouts, use a binder for printed workouts, use a meal plan tracker like My Fitness Pal, track your habits with Fitbit, measure your fat with calipers, use a tape to measure your results and take photos to visually track your progress.

Relax and Love – Show love to yourself and love the world, smile and be friendly, do good deeds and always pass it forward. Learn to meditate, practice deep breathing, take vacations, take long hot baths, get a massage every now and again and learn to release toxic harmful thoughts and beliefs.

Be Punctual – If you are 5 minutes early, you are on time.

If you have to be out from work or school, or if you know you will be tardy, give your employer or teacher at least a 24 hour notice, or whatever the work policy states. An unanticipated tardy always merits a phone call, text, or email, as soon as you realize you will be late.

Be Focused – Keep your eye on the ball: Track your goals, meal plans and vision boards. You will be amazed when you see the forward progress. Set great intentions for yourself and stay focused on them 24/7.

Commit to personal development: Lifestyle and behavior changes are essential for transformation. The body cannot be transformed without challenging the mind and spirit as well.

Be Positive – Celebrate all wins. Fuel your mind with the attitude that will support your success.

Train and develop with a spirit of adventure. An open mind provides opportunities for learning, growth, and Fun!

Absolutely no whining allowed, in whatever you are doing. Feedback is always welcome, but complaints are forbidden.

Be Inspirational – No one gets left behind. It is important to be supportive and encouraging to your friends and colleagues. We are a community of individuals seeking to better ourselves and must lead as well as follow.

Be Respectful to Yourself – Garbage in, garbage out. What you put inside your mind, body and spirit is directly reflected by your condition. It is your responsibility to create a clean space in your life mentally, physically, spiritually, emotionally, and socially.

Stay active. Be committed to an active life.

Be Respectful to Others – Take your turn, share, and clean up after yourself.

Avoid gossip. If you have a problem with someone, it is your responsibility to discuss it directly with that person.

Be Accountable – Stand up for your goals and commitments. Be truthful in your efforts and communication with all others.

For all values, you must be willing to call out others and be called out. If you witness a friend or loved one not living up to mutually agreed upon values, hold them accountable in a loving and respectful way. If you are not in alignment with your values, admit your mistakes and reaffirm your commitment.

About the Author

Fadi Malouf, fitness and performance nutrition specialist, is a body building champion, physical fitness trainer, actor, model, public speaker, and life coach. He has won many international body-building competitions, and has appeared in numerous magazines, including Sports and Fitness, Flex & Natural Health, International Muscle-Mag, Atlanta Sports & Fitness, and Jezebel. He has performed in many televised Bodybuilding competitions, TV commercials and acted in supporting roles in several films. Fadi lives near Atlanta, Georgia, from where he serves as president and proprietor of his own personal fitness and consulting organization.

A Word From Fadi.

Health & Fitness is my life! I was the kid that road his bicycle everywhere, while racing my friends to every stopping point and playing any sports that time allowed! At the young age of seventeen my life as a natural bodybuilder began. Bodybuilding taught me great discipline and understanding of the human body. Today my focus is on balancing my social life, friends, travel, and my fitness life. My health and fitness choices keep me busy at least 6 days a week with 4 days of weight resistance training, a day of core conditioning along with speed and agility training. I also perform yoga and swim at least once a week. Currently my favorite sport is volleyball. I also love to participate in outdoor adventures such as hiking, running, skydiving and racing in the Warrior Dash. I love to play with modern tech toys! The Body by Fadi Virtual Trainer is my preferred and most trusted training platform. I live to play and love to share!

I invite you to train with me and I invite you to become a Body By Fadi member.

What People Say About Fadi:

Nominated Entrepreneur and Fittest Friend of the year in 2011 Fadi Malouf is a lifetime drug-free professional bodybuilder with 19 years of professional experience in the fitness industry. He is regarded as having one of the world's most symmetrical and defined natural physiques and is named one of the best personal trainers is Atlanta.

Fadi is certified through International Sports Sciences Association (ISSA) as a Fitness and Performance Nutritional Specialist. He is equipped to give you direction towards your specific goals and needs. As your trainer he will set up a program designed solely for you through exercise, diet and supplementation. He will help educate and guide you toward a new way of thinking and living. His focus is on your health because your results are his measurement of success. Please feel free to ask him any questions you may have about fitness and achieving a healthy lifestyle.

Find Out More

www.fadimalouf.com

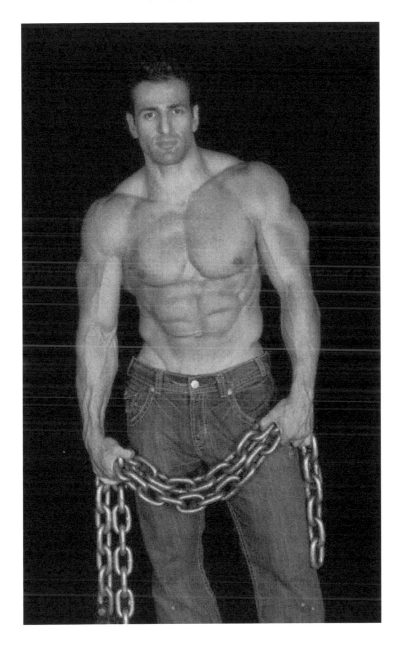

About Body By Fadi

Body by Fadi is a health and fitness company which promotes health education and guidance for clients toward specific goals and needs by setting up programs designed solely for the individual through exercise, nutrition and food supplements.

Now You Can Finally Lose Weight From Any Location with a Personal Trainer on Your Smart Phone, Lap Top, IPad or Computer.

With Body By Fadi's Virtual Trainer You Have a Personal Trainer Everywhere You Go

Workout Anywhere, Anytime
Track Your Weight Loss Progress
24/7 Support From Real Life Personal Trainers

There are many online diet centers available on the Internet today. Almost all of them are designed to respond to the client automatically, based on answers to a series of questions. The responses will place the client into a profile category. Then an auto-responder will forward diets based on the clients category. A person never even looks at the clients data and does not, therefore, have the opportunity to hear the clients "cry for help" when it inevitably arises. That's why Body By Fadi is so unique. Fitness expert Fadi Malouf and one of his Fitness Professionals will review the clients profile personally. Only then are meal planning and exercise programs developed or customized to meet the clients personal health and fitness goals.

Services Offered:
- 6,000 Professional Workout Videos
- Over 750 Pre-Made Workouts
- 465 Professional Fitness Classes
- Custom Workout Programs
- 30, 60, 90 Day Prepackaged Programs
- Competition Programs
- A Personalized Progress Tracker
- Dietary Analysis of Your Daily Eating Habits
- Nutrition Guidance & Custom Meal Planning
- Detox Plans
- Raw Food & Vegan Guidance and Meal Planning
- Body Sculpting / Bodybuilding
- Corrective Exercise
- Weight or Fat Loss
- Weight Gain
- Strength Training
- Flexibility Training
- Functional Training
- Sports Conditioning
- Core Conditioning
- Supplement Plans
- Exercise Routines
- Wellness & Lifestyle Coaching
- Walking Program & Corporate Wellness

Check Us Out

www.fadimalouf.com

Other Titles From Core Keepers Publishing

Currently Available

Living On High Speed by Coach Scott Black
A Raw and Vegan Wellness Guide That Contains Over 200 Blender Recipes.
https://www.createspace.com/4624492

Coming Soon

Body by Fadi
The most comprehensive look at all things wellness which includes workout programs for all 3 body types, ectomorphs / endomorphs and mesomorphs.

The Body By Fadi Tales
Life changing Stories of how each person and different body types in life goes through and over comes difficult trials, self doubts, and destructive relationships.

Endo's Journey
Meso's Journey
Ecto's Journey

The Veil - The Novel
A spiritual thriller that pits one man against the rising tide of demonic oppression and domination.

Made in the USA
Columbia, SC
15 January 2018